An Ethic for Health Promotion

An Ethic for Health Promotion

Rethinking the Sources of Human Well-Being

David R. Buchanan

New York   Oxford
OXFORD UNIVERSITY PRESS
2000

Oxford University Press

Oxford   New York
Athens   Auckland   Bangkok   Bogotá   Buenos Aires   Calcutta
Cape Town   Chennai   Dar es Salaam   Delhi   Florence   Hong Kong   Istanbul
Karachi   Kuala Lumpur   Madrid   Melbourne   Mexico City   Mumbai
Nairobi   Paris   São Paulo   Singapore   Taipei   Tokyo   Toronto   Warsaw

and associated companies in
Berlin   Ibadan

Copyright © 2000 by Oxford University Press, Inc.

Published by Oxford University Press, Inc.,
198 Madison Avenue, New York, New York, 10016
http://www.oup-usa.org

Oxford is a registered trademark of Oxford University Press

Library of Congress Cataloging-in-Publication Data
Buchanan, David Ross.
An ethic for health promotion :
rethinking the sources of human well-being /
David R. Buchanan.
p.   cm.   Includes bibliographical references and index.
ISBN 0-19-513057-X
1. Health promotion—Moral and ethical aspects.
2. Helath promotion—Philosophy.
I. Title.
RA427.8.B83   2000   613'.01—dc21   99-23897

9 8 7 6 5 4 3 2 1

Printed in the United States of America
on acid-free paper

Preface

An Ethic for Health Promotion is an effort to rethink the means and ends of achieving human well-being. The book is divided into two parts. Chapters 1–4 describe the shortcomings and pitfalls of the scientific framework for thinking about the practice of health promotion. The remainder of the book, Chapters 5–9, presents an alternative direction for the field.

The first chapter presents a sketch of the major themes that attest to the need for a new direction for the field of health promotion. The book starts from the premise that the nature of modern public health problems has shifted, and hence their amelioration will require a different approach than the paradigm of power, mastery, and control that has guided the field since the emergence of the modern scientific outlook. Because of their social and behavioral etiology, the leading causes of morbidity and mortality today are inescapably political and ethical issues. The origins of these problems are not well understood, but based on the analysis by the Canadian philosopher Charles Taylor in his *The Malaise of Modernity*, the book examines the rise of instrumental reason as one major source of modern moral malaise. Drug abuse, violence, promiscuous sexuality, the spread of human immunodeficiency virus/acquired immunodeficiency syndrome (HIV/ AIDS), teen pregnancy, infant mortality, obesity, anorexia, smoking, and alcoholism are here seen as symptoms of this underlying malaise. Tragically, the scientific approach to health promotion both reflects and reinforces this modern instrumental outlook. Hence, the dominant approach is not only ill-equipped to alleviate these problems, but it may in fact exacerbate the underlying social conditions that give rise to them in the first place. Based on these concerns, *An Ethic for Health Promotion* advocates for a new direction for the field.

Chapter 2 opens with an overview of current public health challenges in one small city, Holyoke, Massachusetts. This case study serves as a reference point for grounding subsequent discussions, however abstract they may seem at times, in the realities of day-to-day public health practice. To put current public health promotion programs into context, the chapter provides a brief history of health promotion, documenting the decline of infectious diseases and the rise of chronic "lifestyle" diseases. It describes how this transformation in the epidemiological distribution of diseases has shifted the primary locus of attention in the field from controlling the *agent* to controlling the *host,* following the time-honored public health model of agent, host, and environment. The chapter then describes the scientific framework for ameliorating health problems in communities like Holyoke. The prevailing approach is based on scientific explanations of the causes (or risk factors) of disease, which enable program developers to identify strategic intervention points to disrupt the chain of causation. The chapter moves on to review the health goals for the nation, as put forward in the United States Surgeon General's report *Healthy People 2000*, and the plan for achieving these goals. It looks next at the pressure generated by the growth of managed care to develop more effective techniques to change patient behaviors that result in health problems and health care costs. The chapter closes by posing further questions about whether contemporary threats to health are amenable to the same types of scientific interventions that have proven successful in conquering infectious diseases and purifying the environment.

The third chapter lays out the major critique of the standard program of scientific research on health behaviors, examining the epistemological shortcomings and ethical pitfalls of the positivist research agenda. It opens with a brief history of shifts in epistemology (i.e., shifts in our understanding of what counts as valid knowledge), looking at the rise in the power and prestige of the scientific method in the modern era relative to other alternative ways of understanding the human condition. The chapter then turns to a discussion of what makes human beings different, laying the foundations for understanding why health promotion research has failed to produce results comparable to those found in the medical sciences. The principal critique challenges the narrow focus on determining "causes" to the exclusion of questions about the meaning, morality, and purposes of human behavior. A discussion of the ethical pitfalls returns to the point of questioning the instrumental interest in controlling people's behavior and to the ramifications of relying on research methods that cast values outside the scope of rational determinations and conclusions. The ethical and epistemological shortcomings besetting the standard research agenda set the stage for recommending an alternative direction for the field.

To illustrate the ethical pitfalls of the current approach, the fourth chapter details three case studies on the iatrogenic effects of applying three prominent theories now widely used in designing health promotion interventions. The three theories discussed and critiqued are social learning theory, social marketing, and empowerment.

After critiquing current practices in health promotion, the book proposes a positive alternative. The fifth chapter provides a full account of practical reason as an antidote to instrumental reason. A number of definitions of practical reason by prominent philosophers are reviewed and three major characteristics distinguishing practical reason from instrumental reason are presented. The chapter also describes many concrete examples of how the exercise of this faculty of judgment is essential for the field. It concludes with a discussion of the warrants for asserting the validity of value judgments.

Chapter 6 opens a discussion reexamining the goals of health promotion. Well-being is defined here in terms of integrity: gaining greater clarity about values that matter and aspiring to live one's life more closely attuned to those values. In contrast to the idea that health is something that can be produced through technically proficient manipulations (reductions, eliminations) of discrete independent risk factors, the framework presented here argues that well-being is achieved through cultivating certain virtues, or dispositions of character. Cultivating the virtue of mindfulness is essential to the attainment of human well-being, both as a cause and as an essential constituent element in being well. Mindfulness is gaining greater self-knowledge, of becoming more aware of felt desires and putting them into perspective, in terms of the kind of person one aspires to be. The goal of health promotion in this view is to encourage and sustain social practices that foster mindfulness about values that matter, which is essential for promoting human integrity. The chapter concludes with several specific examples of how this framework for thinking about the means and ends of health promotion can be put into practice.

The seventh chapter takes up the question of community well-being. It starts with a synopsis of Michael Sandel's analysis of the sources of our current civic discontents. In his study, modern American discontent is traced to a preoccupation with individual rights to the neglect and disregard of nurturing a sense of belonging, a concern for the whole, and a respect for the social bonds of community. His analysis indicates that the sense of unraveling, the erosion of community, and the loss of self-government felt in modern life stems from the corruption of our political practices, which have increasingly become sheer instrumental, strategic processes for advancing self-interests. On a philosophical level, as confidence in our ability to discern rationally defensible understandings of the common good has waned, we have been drawn increasingly towards the idea that we need stronger procedural protections of individual rights. Parallels are then drawn between Sandel's concerns with the emergence of the "procedural republic" and Taylor's analysis of the rise of instrumental reason. A number of factors contributing to the erosion of trust and social solidarity are reviewed, with particular attention to recent work on the decline of civil society. The role of the virtue of civility in regenerating trust and social solidarity is described. The chapter ends with recommendations regarding the role of health promotion in reviving social practices in civil society.

Chapter 8 presents recommendations for putting the proposed framework for health promotion into practice, focusing on the three linked arenas of research, training, and program development. The opening section discusses the different goals, methods, and assumptions found in humanistic research and their applicability to health promotion. The next part presents an agenda for reframing graduate training programs to promote the use of practical reason and refine ethical sensitivities and sensibilities. The chapter closes with a case study of the El Centro de Educacion, Prevencion, y Educacion (CEPA) project, a community-based HIV/ AIDS prevention program in Holyoke, to illustrate how programs might draw on the principles advanced in this book.

The final chapter proposes that the sources of human well-being lie promoting social practices that enable people to live more closely in tune with the values of justice, caring, and responsibility. Instead of technical efficiency, *An Ethic for Health Promotion* recommends an ethical human relationship of caring as the central value upon which to build the practice of health promotion. The book closes with final reflections on the prospects for putting a new mode of health promotion into practice.

Amherst, Massachusetts   D. R. B.
May 1999

Acknowledgments

I have read hundreds of "acknowledgments" sections, but I have never understood their significance until now. I usually read them for name-dropping, to find out if there are other authors whose work I should be aware of. I never realized how much writing a book depends on the support of friends and colleagues.

A big part of the impetus for writing this book came from feeling the constraints of writing journal articles. I would get feedback asking me to expand on some point, and think, yes, I would love to but it will take another forty pages. I could see the relationship between different pieces that I had written, but the connections were far from obvious (especially, unfortunately, to t & p committees). So, it was time to bring the various pieces together and flesh out some ideas that needed more time and attention. But having a bunch of ideas that seem to be related and getting them down onto paper in coherent fashion is another matter. Two dear friends, Sharry Erzinger and David Powers, read every word of some painful first drafts. Their extensive advice and suggestions has had an immeasurable impact, touching on every page. I am deeply grateful for their help.

I have also benefited from the many thoughtful comments and conversations with a wider sphere of colleagues who took time from their busy schedules to look at different parts. I would like to thank Nina Wallerstein, Allan Steckler, Keith Tones, Bev Ovrebo, Lori Dorfman, Ken McLeory, David Foster, Caroline Wang, Dan Merrigan, and George Cernada. I doubt that I have done justice to Bev's idea that this might represent the "Berkeley School of Thought," but I still like the sound of it and hope others can find the time to do better by it. I would especially like to thank Ron Labonte, who came through with some extremely encouraging words when I sorely needed them. I know how difficult it is to find the time to review an unsolicited manuscript (as I am finding out now with some expectations of reciprocity) and I sincerely appreciate the time they took for me.

I would also like to thank my dear friends in Holyoke who have taught me a lot about community and other ways of doing health promotion. Edna Apostol, Dalila Balfour, Carlos Santiago, Carmen Claudio, and Gladys Lebron made me aware of how deeply instilled the Protestant Ethic is in mainstream American culture and showed me there are other values more important than efficiency. I feel blessed to have had one of those rare magical creative moments in life with them when our work was truly inspired.

I imposed an earlier draft on my students. Class discussions were pointed and lively. Michelle Spaziani, Michael Glantz, Angel Marrero, Michael Scanlon, Beth Donohoe, and Syed Bukhari provided particularly detailed and considerate critiques, challenging me to replace easy rhetoric with reasoned argument. I also thank Katy Ryan for her painstaking diligence in editing the text through each revision.

Finally, a special word of appreciation to two of my teachers, Merry Minkler and Bob Bellah. Their scholarship is a continuing inspiration.

Contents

An Ethic for Health Promotion

"Medicine heals the sicknesses of the body, but wisdom rids the soul of its sufferings."

—Democritus

1

DISQUIETUDES

One day not long ago, the *New York Times* ran three articles that flag the major concerns of this book. The first article, "Clinton Wants Anti-Drug Ads for Youth," described the Clinton administration's proposal to spend $175 million on a national advertising campaign to dissuade teenagers from experimenting with marijuana and other drugs. The second, "Drug and Sex Programs Called Effective in Fight Against AIDS," summarized the release of a National Institutes of Health (NIH) report that decries the intrusion of morality and politics into decisions about implementing sex education and needle exchange programs in local communities. The third article, "Weight Loss From Out of a Bottle," described how weight loss centers are increasingly abandoning a philosophy of sensible eating and increased exercise to prescribe instead a new generation of diet pills to curb overeating.[1] Similar headlines can be found in newspapers across the country on almost any day of the week.

The common theme running through these articles is that science and technology will provide the tools to address our nation's health problems and that politics and morality stand in the way of taking full advantage of these advances. To prevent drug abuse, the executive office proposes to implement a well-financed national media campaign, broadcasting skillfully constructed messages that use the most effective techniques known to the communication sciences. To prevent acquired immunodeficiency syndrome (AIDS), a panel of experts from the NIH recommends stepped up public distribution of sterile syringes and more sex education programs in schools. To reduce obesity (a risk factor for heart disease, the leading cause of death in the nation), researchers have developed new drugs with greater power to control appetite. In short, applied scientific research offers the best prospect for remedying public health problems. It is a tantalizing picture and one that I think fairly represents the consensus of official opinion on how to improve the nation's health.

According to the NIH panel, one major obstacle to alleviating these health problems is the interjection of moral and political compunctions into health policy decisions. The panel sees public objections to needle exchange and sex education programs as foolishly subjecting people to preventable harm. Such moral and political concerns are irrational and unwarranted. Any qualms should be dismissed on the basis of objective, scientific evidence of program effectiveness in reducing infection rates, without producing measurable increases in local drug use or levels of sexual activity. In the eyes of this panel, the evidence is conclusive, further discussion costly.

What are we to make of these articles? How are we to think about improving the health and well-being of individuals and communities? Do the results of scientific research offer the best guide to better living? Are moral apprehensions archaic and unfortunate obstacles? Does it matter whether we lose weight through pills, or through diet and exercise? Or whether teenage drug use is reduced through the same techniques that are used to induce them to start smoking or drink beer? How might these different ways of promoting health make a difference in terms of the quality of outcomes? This text explores these and other related questions.

PURPOSES

The purpose of this book is to advocate a new way of thinking about promoting individual and community well-being. Currently, the field is committed to the development of a science of health promotion. *An Ethic for Health Promotion* argues that the relatively recent emergence of health problems with a largely social and behavioral etiology as the leading causes of morbidity and mortality now makes health promotion[2] an inherently and inescapably ethical and political endeavor. Because the nature of the problems has changed, the future of health promotion will require a different approach than that taken in the past. The ideas presented here are an attempt to fill the void created by an excessive reliance on the scientific method to analyze modern health problems and to design prevention programs.

The problems facing the field of public health today—drug abuse, teen pregnancy, alcoholism, infant mortality, drunk-driving deaths, heart disease, homicide, smoking, AIDS, suicide, child abuse, obesity, domestic violence, strokes, and lack of exercise—are largely attributable to the choices people make, individually and collectively, about how they want to lead their lives.[3] The reasons people might adopt behaviors that harm their own health are not well understood, nor how best to address these problems. This book reviews the work of a number of scholars, largely unknown to the field of public health, who have much to offer in terms of understanding the origins of these modern maladies. The major authors discussed are Charles Taylor, Robert Bellah, Michael Sandel, and Martha Nussbaum, a philosopher, sociologist, political theorist, and classics scholar, respectively. Their thinking poses a thought-provoking alternative to the standard scientific framework now guiding public health promotion research, training, and program development.

In introducing this framework, *An Ethic for Health Promotion* puts forward a new set of concepts and vocabulary. Thinking in the field of health promotion is currently framed by the scientific terminology of morbidity and mortality rates, risk factors, randomized control trials, independent and dependent variables, null hypotheses, cost–benefit analyses, and effective behavior change techniques. This book recommends a new direction marked by the concepts of well-being, integrity, virtues, autonomy, responsibility, civility, caring, and solidarity. These concepts better reflect the larger aims of the field and the direction advocated here. For, as the ethicist Daniel Callahan once remarked, how we think about questions and the way we frame the issues usually make all the difference in people's lives.[4]

In presenting the work of these scholars, I am going to convey a message that may make many colleagues uncomfortable. This book is critical of the unstinting institutional commitment to the positivist (experimental) paradigm of scientific research for determining the causes of "lifestyle" diseases and for developing interventions to prevent them. This commitment is most conspicuously evident in the research protocols of the National Institutes of Health, which provide the principal funding for research that sets the standards for program development. This research is directed at the development of a science of health promotion copied exactly on the model used in the biomedical sciences, with the explicit purpose of producing more effective techniques for modifying people's behaviors. This book explains why this approach is wrong headed, both ethically and epistemologically. Indeed, in the view of the authors cited above, not only is the current framework for thinking about contemporary ills unlikely to resolve them, it is in fact exacerbating the very conditions that give rise to them in the first place.

An Ethic for Health Promotion provides the philosophical foundations for a different type of practice in the field. A dissident stream of researchers and practitioners has periodically challenged the idea that the mission of health education is to change individual behavior,[5] but these views have had little impact on federal research priorities, government planning documents, or the allocation of program dollars. This book presents a sound, defensible alternative to the quest for a science of human promotion. Many people practice a far different approach to health promotion that cannot be squared with the technical scientific framework; their work affirms the values of autonomy, justice, caring, and solidarity over the pursuit of more effective behavior change techniques. This book explains why this alternative tradition is better suited to realizing human well-being and provides the philosophical basis for its justification. Instead of scientific reasoning, the alternative proposed here is based on practical reasoning. Instead of seeking the power to change people's behavior, it recommends seeking common understandings with community members about the good life for human beings. Instead of pursuing the development of a science of health promotion, it recommends an ethical and political process of improving institutional practices in order to foster individual and community well-being.

The premise of this book can be stated in three interlocking propositions:

- The kinds of health problems now facing the field have shifted, but our thinking about how to respond to them has not shifted accordingly. The leading health problems of the day have shifted from infectious diseases to chronic "lifestyle" diseases. The locus of responsibility has thus shifted from invasive microorganisms to human volitions, but the framework for thinking about how to deal with these problems has not changed. It is still a paradigm of power, mastery, and control.

- The source of most major health problems in industrialized nations today lies in the choices people make about how to lead their lives, but human choices are inextricably linked to understandings about how people ought to lead their lives. The increasing significance of human volitions in modern health problems takes us inexorably into the realm of ethical and political concerns. The question "How should one live?" is the classical starting point for all ethical inquiry. Yet, the scientific method is incapable of providing answers to normative questions: questions about the validity of different human values, the significance of different visions of the good life for human beings, and the quality of different ideals about how we think we should live.

- The strength of the scientific method lies in its ability to predict and control outcomes, but when the outcome of interest is human behavior, the commitment to the scientific method undermines the most fundamental understandings of ethical human relationships. The scientific method attempts to test and prove cause-and-effect relationships. These relationships are ideally and most conclusively verified through conducting experiments that predict and produce changes in the dependent variable of interest. The power to control outcomes is thus an inherent byproduct of testing hypotheses in any experimental research design. The commitment to the scientific method thus sanctions the idea that the purpose of health promotion is to seek and to wield the power necessary to produce changes in people's behaviors. This book contests the propriety of this goal.

The field of health promotion needs to revive and reorient its practices toward bringing people together as citizens and community members to decide for themselves the kinds of lives they think are most worth living, rather than continuing to develop the "technologies of prevention."[6] Explaining the shortcomings of the current approach and establishing the foundations for an alternative approach will take us into complex philosophical issues, but we ignore them at our peril. As the sociologist Todd Gitlan recently put it, "You may not be interested in philosophy, but philosophy is interested in you. . . . People think within the intellectual and cultural currents that surround them—currents with histories, even if the sources cannot be seen from downstream."[7] The lack of philosophical training among social scientists in general has been lamented;[8] the problem is probably even greater for behavioral scientists in the health field, due to their proximity, allegiance, and perhaps envy of the successes of medical science. But greater familiarity with the ethical and epistemological assumptions underlying current practices and with the merits of an alternative approach is essential in order to establish a more propitious and principled ethic for health promotion.

CHALLENGES

A number of considerations indicate that a new direction for the field of health promotion is now in order. I want to start by briefly reviewing several recent summaries regarding the state of American society. These works introduce the challenges we now face and present us with questions about the roots of our current health problems. Then I suggest that standard social scientific explanations have not taken us very far in understanding the nature of modern health issues, specifically those with a social and behavioral etiology. These explanations seem particularly meager when compared to the results of research in the medical sciences. In addition, I find scant evidence that scientifically designed interventions have been effective in preventing modern health problems. On the contrary, all evidence indicates that the activities that have helped people most are those that have evolved out of a philosophy of self-help, mutual support, and communal solidarity.

While the state of American society does not lend itself to easy summarization and conflicting data are always at hand, a variety of sources and evidence point to some disturbing trends. Interestingly, representatives from across the political spectrum have come to similar conclusions about the significance of these figures.

In the middle of the road, Derek Bok, former president of Harvard University, provides an ambitious analysis in his *The State of the Nation* (1996). He introduces his book with the following observations. In opinion poll data solicited in April 1995, 74% of Americans declared themselves "dissatisfied with the way things are going in this country." Similarly, in 1994, more than 50 percent of the American people felt their children would not have as good a life as they themselves had enjoyed. That same year, the Harris Alienation Index, a measure of how far the public feels estranged from the powers that be, climbed to a record high. As Bok summed up the mood of the country at the time of the 1996 presidential election, "By every available measure, ordinary citizens had lost confidence in the major institutions of the country and in the leaders responsible for its welfare."[9]

Representing the liberal left, Marc Miringoff of the Fordham Institute for Innovation in Social Policy has been compiling an Index of Social Health for the past 10 years.[10] The Index is a composite catalogue of 16 different measures, ranging from straightforward health indicators (e.g., infant mortality, teen suicide, drug abuse, drunk-driving deaths, homicide) to broader social indices (e.g., the number of children in poverty, the income gap between the rich and the poor, the number of high school dropouts). Indicators were carefully selected to include measures for all age groups: children, youth, adults, and the elderly.

With data going back to 1970, the Index of Social Health reached its highest point—77.5 on a scale of 100—in 1973. It has declined consistently since that time, reaching its nadir in 1994. (See Fig. 1–1.) Four out of the worst five years occurred between 1990 and 1995. As Miringoff summarizes, "Overall, since 1970, America's social health declined from 74 in 1970 to 37 in 1994, dropping 49 percent. During that time, 11 problems worsened and 5 improved. This pattern of decline involves Americans across the age spectrum. . . . The worsening of so many social problems carries adverse implications for the social fabric of the country. So significant a decline in our society's ability to cope with its social problems may well help to explain the sense of unease felt by so many Americans today."[11]

On the conservative side, William Bennett, former Secretary of Education, Director of the Office of National Drug Control Policy, and Chair of the National Endowment for the Humanities, has contributed a "report card" on the state of American society. In the *Index of Leading Cultural Indicators* (1994), Bennett has drawn together hundreds of charts, graphs, and tables documenting America's sociocultural condition. The indicators are grouped into five categories: (*1*) crime, (*2*) family and children (out-of-wedlock births, divorce, abortion, etc.), (*3*) youth (teen pregnancy, teen suicide, etc.), (*4*) education (levels of achievement, problems in school, etc.), and (*5*) popular culture (amount of television viewing, its content, church attendance, etc.). Illustrative of the major findings, since 1960, violent crime has increased by 560%; the number of unmarried pregnant teenagers has nearly doubled; teen suicide has increased by more than 200%; and, the number of divorces has increased nearly 200%, while the marriage rate is at an all-time low. The list goes on, but the message remains the same.

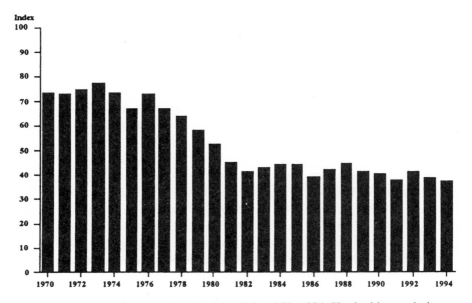

Figure 1–1. Index of Social Health of the U.S., 1970–1994. Used with permission, Miringoff, *Index of Social Health*, (1996).

Bennett concludes, "According to the findings in this book, in many ways the condition of America is not good. Over the past 3 decades we have experienced substantial social regression. Today the forces of social decomposition are challenging—and in some instances, overtaking—the forces of social composition. And when decomposition takes hold, it exacts an enormous human cost."[12]

Finally, a group of social scientists, laying claim to an impartial, objective assessment, has weighed in on the subject too. Striving to provide a jargon-free guide to correct the often misleading, partial, and erroneous information reaching the American public, this team of researchers, led by Urie Bronfenbrenner, the prominent psychologist and professor of Human Development at Cornell University, has compiled and analyzed data on issues quite like the preceding indices, although their report also includes data on more intangible issues, such as questions of moral integrity. Their categories cover youth, crime, the economy, families, poverty, education, and age. The emerging statistical profile, especially with regard to youth, underscores current threats to America's well-being.

For example, the authors report that, in national survey data, the percentage of high school students who said they had cheated on exams doubled—from 34% to 68%—between 1969 and 1989. Similarly, while in 1975, 35% of high school seniors agreed that "most people can be trusted," by 1992, that number had dropped to 18%. At the same time, weekly church attendance declined from 44% in 1980 to 30% in 1990. In 1990, 31.5% of male high school students reported having carried a weapon to school in the previous month.

In their conclusion, Bronfenbrenner and his colleagues see two sets of problems now facing American society. The first is economic, centering on rising inequality and the falling standard of living for the poor. The second set of problems they find more difficult to characterize: "Falling wages and lagging growth are well-defined phenomena; a 'decline in values' is not. But the vagueness of the problem in no way undermines the urgency of the concern. Something is terribly wrong."[13]

To wrap up, in a study we will return to later in greater depth, the political philosopher and Professor of Government at Harvard, Michael Sandel, offers a succinct synopsis of our current discontents: "One is the fear that, individually and collectively, we are losing control of the forces that govern our lives. The other is the sense that, from family to neighborhood to nation, the moral fabric of the community is unraveling around us. These two fears—for the loss of self-government and the erosion of community—together define the anxiety of the age."[14]

Based on these diverse statistical portraits, collected by parties with different backgrounds and different agenda, a picture is beginning to emerge of contemporary threats to health. Without wishing to fall into the old trap of millennial doomsaying, I offer this brief sketch to indicate the kinds of challenges the field of health promotion must now take up. To return to questions posed at the outset, to what can we attribute the emergence of these threats to our health and well-being?

A key tenet of the field of health promotion today is that health problems are attributable to the prevalence and distribution of identifiable risk factors and that the most fruitful approach for identifying suspect risk factors is scientific research. The scientific method is regarded as having indisputable superiority in determining the causes of these problems. The purpose of such research is to identify the underlying social and psychological factors that cause people to behave in ways that compromise their health (i.e., to start smoking, to take drugs, to overeat, to commit violent acts, etc.). In light of the significant accomplishments of science, from heart bypass surgery to landing men on the moon, one might expect similarly striking progress through these methods in identifying the causes of and solutions to contemporary health problems.

But the current program of health promotion research has not produced a cogent response to questions about causation. As we shall see, because health has both physical and social dimensions, understanding the nature of modern ailments presents new problems that are not readily amenable to scientific analysis. For now, in surveying the field, it is simply an indisputable fact that studies of behavioral health problems have not been able to produce results even remotely comparable to those found in biomedical research.

To illustrate, Figure 1–2 provides one example taken from a well-regarded study of the initiation of youthful drug use.[15] It demonstrates the proliferation of variables typically found in health promotion research these days. The researchers identified a large number of different factors with statistically significant relationships to the dependent variable of interest, the onset of teenage drug use. All were also found to have complex feedback relationships with one another—meaning that "effects" were found to have an impact on their own "causes." Unlike the parsimonious laws found in the natural sciences, we find here instead a complicated picture depicting an indefinite expansion in the number of independent variables and the absence of clear, unidirectional, cause-precedes-effect relationships. The picture becomes even more complicated when one learns that the sum total of all these factors still accounts for only a small fraction of the variance in behavior. So, despite the attempts to explain behavior by adding more variables into the equation, this accumulation does not enable one to predict very well whether or not someone will start taking drugs. Further complicating matters, the identified variables stand only in a "probabilistic" relationship to one another. That is, social variables have not been found to cause outcomes in constant manner (unlike, say, gravity, which is uniform throughout the known universe), but only make any given outcome more likely.

Two additional considerations provide further support for reconsidering the current direction of the field. First, a growing mass of evidence shows that the most carefully designed scientific interventions intended to reduce modern health problems have not proven successful. Carefully controlled, scientifically designed

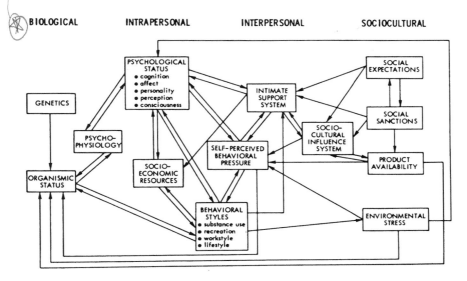

Figure 1–2. Interactive theory of drug use. National Institute on Drug Abuse (1980).

health promotion interventions—such as the many heart disease prevention programs[16] (the Stanford three- and five-community studies,[17] the Minnesota Heart Health plan,[18] the Pawtucket trials,[19] the Karelia intervention[20]), the highly intensive and individualized Multiple Risk Factor Intervention Trials[21] (MRFIT), and the more recent National Cancer Institute (NCI)-sponsored smoking reduction plan, the Community Intervention Trial[22] (COMMIT)—have produced little evidence of success. In reviewing the results of these many large scale randomized control trials, even ardent advocates of the science of health promotion acknowledge that they have produced "disappointing results."[23]

Finally, in direct contrast, there are ample indications that the most beneficial responses to these problems have come from people acting on their own without recourse to scientifically designed interventions. The most effective treatment for alcohol abuse is Alcoholics Anonymous (AA).[24] The most effective treatment for substance abuse is an analogous 12-step program based on the AA model.[25] Likewise, we know that 90% of people who quit smoking successfully do so on their own without the assistance of professional interventions.[26] The most successful method of weight reduction is, again, self-help groups.[27] And the decline in infection rates in the AIDS epidemic, especially among gay men, is widely attributed to a groundswell of nonprofessional community activism, and not to replication and dissemination of scientifically proven interventions.[28]

These observations have led me to the conclusion that it is time to consider a new direction for the field.

THE SOURCES OF MODERN MALAISE

If we accept that health problems with a social and behavioral etiology are the most significant challenges confronting the field today, that scientific interventions have not been shown to be effective in their amelioration, and that the source of these problems may lie in a collective sense of "alienation," "social decomposition," "a decline in values," and an "unraveling of the moral fabric," it may be worthwhile to consider what scholars in other fields are saying about the sources of our current troubles.

In *The Malaise of Modernity* (1992), the preeminent Canadian philosopher Charles Taylor analyzes the origins of modern malaise, identifying "the dark side of individualism" and "the primacy of instrumental reason" as the two principal sources.[29] The pages that follow focus on the issue of instrumental reason. As Taylor defines it, "By 'instrumental reason,' I mean the kind of rationality we draw on when we calculate the most economical applications of means to a given end. Maximum efficiency, the best cost–output ratio, is its measure of success."[30] There are undoubtedly other factors contributing to the development of contemporary social health problems, but as this book shows, understanding the influence of instrumental reason is essential for understanding one of the most important underlying sources of current threats to health. Even more pertinent to my concerns, the quest for a science of health promotion both reproduces and reinforces the instrumental outlook that Taylor and others see at the core of our modern moral malaise.

Taylor sees the growing recourse to instrumental reason as a "massively important phenomenon" underlying the perplexing sense of loss, decline, and disintegration widely felt in modern culture. Succinctly stated, instrumental reason is the intellectual tendency to give precedence to thinking about means, rather than ends. Coined by the seminal German sociologist Max Weber, the term "instrumental reason" refers to a pattern of thinking dedicated to the methodical expansion of human dominion "by means of an increasingly precise calculation of adequate means."[31] Weber used the term to characterize the modern preoccupation with determining the most effective means to a given end, to the neglect and detriment of the evaluation of the ends themselves. As the sociologist Philip Selznick states, "Reason is instrumental when it abdicates responsibility for determining ends and restricts itself to ways and means."[32]

In laying out the concept of "instrumental reason" (*Zweckrationalitaet*), Weber was trying to identify and define the fundamental driving force behind the distinctive pattern of modernization that evolved in the West. Weber developed this protean idea in an effort to explain why Western civilization progressed the way it did and why it differed from the direction other civilizations took. In contrast to Marx's focus on material conditions, Weber saw the process of modernization in the West driven by the emergence of a certain, distinct form of consciousness: a characteristic "worldview," "attitude," and "way of life." With the rise and spread of the Protestant Ethic, he found the main engine of modernization in the West to be the emergence of an ethos of world mastery.[33]

Weber traces the origins of this distinctive ethos back to the Reformation, emerging at the dawn of the sixteenth century in response to the pressures generated by the ideas of Luther and Calvin. The seeds of this "specific and peculiar rationalism"[34] took root in their revelation of a new ascetic calling to master the environment, which then meshed with the emergence of a new empirical experimental science. These twin pillars grew in significance because they solved the Calvinist need for certainty about salvation. Since a mystical union with an absolutely transcendental deity was no longer permissible, believers could no longer aspire to be a vessel of God, but had to think of themselves instead as a tool of the divine will. Prosperity, reaped through taming and subjugating the environment, came to be seen as a sign of serving God's glory. At the same time, with the growing success of the scientific method in gaining control over the natural world, scientific knowledge promised an end to the presumptuous illusions of sinful man, those false "idols of the mind," as the father of modern science, Francis Bacon, called them.

The rise of instrumental reason is the central theme unifying the whole of Weber's work. In Weber's distinctive methodological style, instrumental reason is an "ideal type" and stands in contrast to "value rationality" (*Wertrationalitaet*).[35] In surveying the full range of Weber's work, Rogers Brubaker identifies four characteristics that distinguish instrumental reason: (*1*) the depersonalization of social relationships, (*2*) the refinement of the techniques of calculation, (*3*) the enhancement of the social importance of specialized knowledge, and (*4*) the extension of technically rationally control over both natural and social processes.[36] Other descriptions of instrumental reason include the intellectual tendency to favor calculation, predictability, precision, specialization, rigor, quantification, standardization, systemization, formal procedures, technique, proficiency, strategic orientation, cost-effectiveness, and the maximization of efficiency over other thought processes.

For Weber, the advance of instrumental reason has bequeathed a deeply ambiguous legacy. It has simultaneously made possible the most distinguishing accomplishments of the modern world and brought about conditions that call into question the entire idea of progress. The paradox arises because, as the sphere of dominance and control has expanded, life appears to have become increasingly meaningless, lacking in moral direction, and dominated by bureaucratic imperatives. The concept of instrumental reason captures his deepest concerns with the problematic nature of the whole of modern life. In his most renowned passages, the ascent of instrumental reason has ushered in an "age of disenchantment" and the "iron cage" of modernity. For Weber, it was a "tragedy of culture," a tragedy represented by the contradiction between "the basic demand that life and the world have a coherent overall meaning and the increasingly evident impossibility of determining this meaning scientifically."[37] We know more and more about determining the means to an end, but less and less about distinguishing which ends are worth pursuing. Science can explain the world by making it predictable, but it cannot help us find purpose in life. It can tell us how to live longer, but not why we should want to do so. With the rise of instrumental reason, the search for causes has vitiated the search for meaning.

The philosopher Charles Larmore summarizes its impact:

> Modern thought, according to Weber, is characterized by an increasingly 'disenchanted' view of the world. In earlier times the ultimate purposes of life were seen as part of the fabric of the world, as part of the Greek 'cosmos' or of Christian 'creation'; the description of fact and the affirmation of norms were not sharply distinguished. The modern era, by contrast, has recast rationality as simply the calculation of efficient means to given ends. This narrower, instrumental conception of reason was what, in Weber's eyes, brought about the unprecedented increase in knowledge and power, prediction and control, characteristic of modern science. But it has meant that ultimate purposes, and the good and the beautiful generally, have come to seem a matter of merely subjective conviction. For Weber, this development was as unstoppable as it was terrifying.[38]

In contrast to instrumental reason, Weber described another type of reasoning process that he called "value rationality" (which, for purposes of consistency, will hereafter referred to as "practical reason"). Building on Weber's work (and a distinction originally made by Aristotle), Taylor and others see a compelling need for reviving the exercise of "practical reason" to counterbalance the bias of instrumental reason. Practical reason addresses questions about the good for human beings. It is reflection on the goals, values, and purposes of human action. It is the thinking process involved in evaluating the quality of the ideals we seek to realize in this life. Practical reason is the exercise of one's critical faculty of judgment in making qualitative distinctions of worth among different goals and choosing one course of action over another in light of the highest good people hope to realize.[39]

In this text, I draw out the contrasts between these different types of reasoning processes as sharply as possible so that we can better see the issues at stake. But it is important to remember that these distinctions are Weberian ideal types. Like all ideal types, there is a complex mixture of these different ways of thinking in real life. Some authors have suggested that they might best be thought of as marking polar ends of a continuum.[40] Defining them as ideal types allows us to see their differences, but in practice there is often an intricate interplay between them.

That said, Weber believed that the burgeoning disposition toward instrumental reasoning would undermine and ultimately nullify the pursuit of practical reason. Testing hypotheses to determine cause-and-effect relationships is the epitome of instrumental means–ends rationality. Yet with the undeniable success of experimental science, many people have come to believe that truth can best be determined by following the procedures defined by the scientific method. Starting with Francis Bacon in the 1500s and culminating in the philosophy of Logical Positivism in the twentieth century, powerfully influential currents of thought have propagated the idea that one can make claims about the truth of any statement if and only if it can be verified through the testing of hypotheses. Conversely, if one cannot verify a statement through these procedures, then it is strictly a matter of subjective convictions and personal preferences. Here is the critical point. Since one cannot test hypotheses about the validity of value statements, value claims have come to be regarded as expressions of subjective opinion and not as "objective" knowledge.[41]

Taylor considers this a colossal categorical mistake. We have confused "the question of what something *is*" with "the question of how it is *known*."[42] That is, just because the validity of value statements cannot be determined by testing hypotheses, that does not mean that values cannot be considered rational, objective, and matters about which we can attain valid knowledge. Against the press of the positivist paradigm, the concern of these scholars is to move beyond the idea that values are nothing more than subjective expressions of personal preferences. Nevertheless, that has been the drift of the modern cast of mind ("Well, that's *your* opinion and everyone is entitled to their own opinion"), which they see lying at the heart of our modern malaise. In Taylor's words, "When one sees that no rational headway can be made in this way in discerning the good, one falls into skepticism and despair."[43]

Eclipsed by the power and prestige now attached to the positivist experimental method, the decline of practical reason has reached the point where we no longer even ask questions about the good for human beings. As the professor of political science Charles Anderson notes, "Scientific empiricism does rather drastically narrow the range of legitimate intellectual concerns. In the contemporary university, one quickly learns that certain questions are out of order. One does not ask persistently about what ought to be done, for normative questions entail what are called value judgments, and these are said to be beyond the scope of scientific analysis."[44] And so finally, in the clash of these different types of reasoning processes, Taylor summarizes the triumph of instrumental reason in the modern era: "Reason is no longer defined substantively, in terms of a vision of the cosmic order, but [only] formally, in terms of the procedures thought ought to follow."[45]

IS THE QUEST FOR A SCIENCE OF HEALTH PROMOTION CONTRIBUTING TO THE PROBLEM?

In health promotion, research is instrumental to the extent that it focuses on identifying the causes of behavior—ascertained through rigorous adherence to well-known and well-defined research methods—and disregards questions about what makes human behavior good. Reflecting the pressures for precision, quantification, and efficiency maximization of these times, the nation's public health goals and objectives are now defined in terms of reducing morbidity and mortality rates.[46] The leading causes of morbidity and mortality are now most influenced by smoking, a poor diet, and lack of exercise. Therefore, health promotion research and practice focus virtually exclusively on developing more effective and efficient means to accomplish these behavioral change objectives. These narrow objectives are indicative of the failure to think through the ends of health promotion.

To press the point about the need for reviving the exercise of practical reason— the type of thinking that asks, "Are the postulated ends worth pursuing, in light of the means they seem to require? Are the institution's values, as presently formulated, worthy of realization? What costs are imposed on *other* ends and *other* values?"[47]—let me be heretical: I do not think that lowering heart disease rates is the most important goal of health promotion. On the contrary, I think most people are drawn to the field because they want to be part of forging social and political conditions in which we all can live together decently.[48] Nonsmoking, a strict diet, and regular exercise are really rather trivial parts of any broader understanding of social well-being, but that is where all of the field's resources are now directed.

A few examples will serve to illustrate the instrumental orientation of the field. It is not my intention to denigrate either the motives or the work of the authors cited. On the contrary, the point is that all of us—public health professionals and society as a whole—are caught up in the larger intellectual currents of these times. In their widely acclaimed text, *Health Behavior and Health Education: Theory, Research, and Practice* (with a newly revised edition released in 1997), the editors Karen Glanz, Frances Lewis, and Barbara Rimer state that the "dominant paradigm" in health promotion and education is "logical positivism," which they strongly endorse.[49] Despite their allegiance, they are not unaware of the potential problems this commitment poses. To their credit, in a significant revision of the first edition of their text, the editors note in passing, "Nevertheless . . . the inherent exercise of power [in developing techniques to effect behavior change] remains a problem."[50] Unfortunately, the ethical dilemma posed by the commitment to the positivist perspective is left unexplored and unresolved.

Consistent with the positivist/instrumental outlook, the introductory chapters are replete with references to maximizing the effectiveness of the means of health promotion. The authors cite "the importance of effective approaches to health-related behavior change" (p. xvi); "theories of health behavior identify targets for change and the methods for accomplishing these changes" (p. xvii); the text's "main purpose: to advance the science of health promotion and education" (p. xvii); "behavioral interventions may grow in importance under managed care when their cost-effectiveness is demonstrated" (p. 6); health education aims at "bringing about behavioral changes in individuals, groups, and larger populations" (p. 7); "the identification of personal and environmental leverage points" (p. 8); "The central concern of health promotion and health education is health behavior. It is . . . the crucial dependent variable in most research" (p. 9); "research programs have been established to identify and test the most effective methods for achieving individual behavioral change" (p. 12); "randomized control trials are the most rigorous test of health behavior interventions" (p. 14); "the search for truth and for an ultimate understanding of the forces that make humans think, feel, and act as they do is the long-term goal" (p. 20); "theories and models *explain* behavior and suggest ways to achieve behavior *change*" (p. 23, emphasis in original); theories "guide the search for modifiable factors" (p. 23); health promotion and health education are concerned with "how to bring about change" and "devoted to developing techniques that change behavior" (p. 26); "theory must meet basic standards for adequacy of research" (p. 28); and, theories for inclusion were selected on the basis of "substantial empirical evidence supporting the theory's validity in predicting or changing health behavior" (p. 28). In summary, they state, "As science and technology advance, the least conquered force of nature remains the human being and his actions and human experiences."[51] This outlook, I submit, is highly instrumental.

In a recent article appearing in one of the field's leading professional journals, the professor of health education Christine Jackson declares, "The value of health education practice lies in its effectiveness . . . behavioral science theories constitute the best available information on why people behave the way they do and practitioners aiming to change health-related behavior would do well to take advantage of this information. More specifically, behavioral science theories identify several attributes of individuals and their surroundings that are causally related to behavior, and thus, theories can guide practitioners' selection of psychological, behavioral, social, and environmental targets for intervention . . . and by doing so increase the likelihood that the program will effect behavior change."[52]

To take another example, on February 20, 1998, the National Institute on Drug Abuse released a Request for Applications (RFA) soliciting research "to inform the National Youth Anti-Drug Media Campaign sponsored by the Office of National Drug Control Policy."[53] The RFA provides funding for "research targeting the full spectrum of settings, from communications research in the laboratory to studies examining the elements and impact of mass media and applied studies using prevention communications in the community." The announcement continues, "Current research suggests that the use of strategies such as indirect influence techniques, conditioning in low-thought situations, and strengthening of existing attitudes show promise for drug prevention programming. However, it is not known if these strategies are universally effective." Further research is necessary to investigate "the role of effective communication as a determinant of intervention success" and "the most effective use of the mass media for reaching all audiences." As a result, "research on effective message construction and delivery in group settings may lead to more cost-effective programs."

These statements well represent the prevailing view with respect to the linked processes of research, practice, and professional preparation in health promotion. Using the same methods as the biomedical sciences, health promotion researchers are seeking the same power to effect targeted outcomes. The premier goal is to eliminate modern threats to health in the same way that an infectious disease like smallpox was eliminated: by discovering the antecedent causes of "lifestyle" diseases; developing and testing interventions that will interrupt, control, or eradicate these causes; and thus, preventing the outbreak. But now the significant difference is that the underlying causes lie primarily in human volitions.

I have three concerns. First, on some level, people who smoke, drink, eat a fatty diet, get pregnant as teenagers, take drugs, or fail to exercise do not share the goals of eliminating smoking, drug-taking, eating red meat, physical inactivity, premarital sex, and so on. They do not share or agree with our vision of how we think they ought to live. However we in the field of health promotion try to rationalize our efforts, we are saying that we think we know how people should live their lives better than they do themselves. And the best way to accomplish our goals is to develop and to wield effective techniques to change their behavior. (To anticipate ready objections, I take up the question of voluntary consent below.)

Second, as we shall see in the next chapter, the research protocols of the National Institutes of Health are designed to uncover the same power to effectively control human behavior that we have already discovered to effectively control high blood pressure. If successful, such discoveries would pose serious threats to human autonomy, dignity, and responsibility. If autonomy, dignity, and responsibility are intrinsic to human well-being, then the current direction of the field is self-defeating.

Third, health promotion research is not now aimed at clarifying normative values, which might prove helpful in assisting people to exercise better judgment. The origins of contemporary health problems, I believe, do indeed lie in disturbances in people's values and judgments about their immediate felt desires. But the scientific method of testing hypotheses is incapable of answering questions about which values should matter to us and why, about the kinds of lives most worth living and the kind of society we should work toward creating together. The abdication of responsibility for pursuing questions about the worthiness of different values is part and parcel of the atrophy, erosion, and decline in values that many scholars see at the core of our current troubles.

Before going any further, I want to carefully restrict the scope of criticism of the scientific approach to health promotion presented in these pages. This critique is not directed at science in general, nor at empirical research, but focuses specifically on the tenets of logical positivism as they are applied to the study of human behavior in health promotion research. As noted above, the editors of the most widely used textbook in the field state unequivocally that the dominant paradigm in health promotion research is logical positivism. Positivists claim that one can determine the validity of a statement if and only if it can be tested empirically, an axiom known as the verification principle.[54] It is this doctrine which this book challenges.

Let me be clear: I think hypothesis testing works remarkably well in the natural sciences, such as physics, chemistry, and medicine. There are variants of "postmodern deconstructionist discourses" in academia that attack the idea of science as a whole. That is not a position put forward here. On the contrary, I think experimental research designs are effective in discovering and demonstrating causal relationships in the natural world, including, notably, the physiological processes of the human body.

Just as the natural sciences are not wholly subsumed by experimental methods (for example, research in geology and ecology), not all research in health promotion involves experimental research designs. In practice, a great deal of research in the field involves simple empiricism. Researchers simply count things (no matter how sophisticated the statistical techniques) and try to see what goes together with what ("correlations"). This text does not question the value of empirical research, although it argues that many of the most important issues now confronting the field cannot be reduced to strictly empirical questions. (Values, for example, are not wholly empirical; they are, in essence, normative phenomena. Beyond what is, they entail creative imaginings of what ought to be. Hence, they can never be completely captured through empirical methods and attempts to do so are usually abysmally reductionistic and distortive.[55]) Likewise, on occasion, when there has been open public debate and a reasonable degree of consensus over the means and ends of a social intervention (e.g., funding Head Start to improve academic achievement, or raising taxes to reduce teen smoking), there is a natural interest in learning whether such policy changes produce the desired outcomes. Quasi-experimental research designs have a valuable role to play in informing public discussions about the merits of continuing such policies.

Although correlational and quasi-experimental research designs are common, the experimental method of hypothesis-testing is a tremendously powerful ideal that guides the bulk of day-to-day research activities in public health, especially research sponsored by the National Institutes of Health (NIH). Randomized control trials are the highest standard against which all other types of research are compared and the endpoint toward which all health research is expected to progress. One major purpose of this book is to show how the commitment to this particular method has displaced other types of research in ways that are ultimately debilitating to the field.

Outside of public health, debates about the status of the social sciences have long been waged.[56] While many social scientists have accepted the idea that the study of the human condition poses unique challenges that are not amenable to the methods used in the natural sciences, I see little evidence that these arguments have had any impact on the research protocols approved by the NIH, nor much acceptance in the field's mainstream research journals.[57] And indeed, because the physiological processes of the human body have been so successfully analyzed using standard scientific hypothesis-testing research methodologies, it is under-standable that calls for "humanistic" approaches to the study of human health should be met with skepticism. But it is precisely because of the unflinching in-stitutional commitment to the positivist perspective in health research that I feel it necessary to present the shortcomings and pitfalls of the positivist methodology as starkly as possible. While many colleagues might argue that a "we-need-both-kinds" position would be less controversial, I believe such a concession would merely allow researchers to carry on complacently with the current research agenda, when I see the instrumental interest in controlling people's behavior as a big part of the problem.

To summarize, I want to acknowledge that (*1*) there are many influences con-tributing to the rise of instrumental reasoning beyond positivist scientific research,[58] (*2*) positivism is one manifestation of the larger cultural phenomenon but not all scientific research is positivist, and (3) not all research in health promotion is positivist although it is the dominant type. Where positivist research in health promotion is consistent with the larger cultural trend toward instrumental reasoning, it suffers from these influences as much as it propagates them. While critical of the current direction of the field, I am not arguing that positivist research in health promotion alone is responsible for all that ails us today. In failing to challenge the larger cultural drift, the "dominant paradigm" in health promotion simply makes things worse, instead of better. With these qualifications in mind, we can conclude the discussion of the ways in which the quest for a science of health promotion both reproduces and reinforces the characteristic modern ethos of striving to extend technical control over both natural and social processes.

Based on what the positivist, hypothesis-testing methodology can and cannot do, instead of strengthening our collective capacity to think more clearly, carefully, and conscientiously about values that matter, the instrumental orientation of health promotion today is headed in the opposite direction. If the field achieved its own stated objectives to gain the power to effectively change human behavior, it would further erode the grounds of human dignity, the individual sense of responsibility, and the most basic understandings of ethical human relationships. We believe human beings have dignity and deserve to be treated with respect because we believe human beings have autonomy, that is, because we believe human beings have a capacity for free choice unlike any other creature on earth. It is autonomy per se which affords humankind its peculiar dignity.[59] Moreover, our entire understanding of the concept of responsibility is anchored in understandings of human beings as free and autonomous agents. If people did not have the capacity to make free choices, then we could not hold them responsible for their actions.

So, in health promotion, whenever we treat people as if we know what they need better than they do themselves and whenever we assume that their behavior is caused or conditioned by antecedent factors (which tacitly sanctions the right to intervene, since they are evidently not fully responsible for the choices they make), we treat them as a means to serve our ends. The fundamental moral principle imperiled by the current direction of the field was originally articulated by Immanuel Kant: "Act so that you treat humanity, whether in your own person or that of another, always as an end and never as a means only." Selznick brings home the point: "The claims of efficiency are strong, but they cannot justify practices that reduce human beings to 'means only.' Such practices make them victims of domination."[60] Or, as Glanz, Lewis, and Rimer remind us, "the inherent exercise of power remains a problem."

One final point—the question of consent and coercion—needs to be addressed before getting into the substance of these matters. Although we will come back to this issue in later chapters, I need to address the question briefly now because it speaks to immediate objections that may be prompted by these introductory remarks.

The standard response to concerns about coercion and manipulation is to invoke voluntary participation. Because the exercise of power over people is inherently problematic, the field of health promotion now relies on an externally superimposed code of ethics. Ethical safeguards to prevent the coercion and manipulation of people are enforced through compliance with a code of standards mandating informed consent and voluntary participation ("ethical cleansing agents," in the memorable words of Duncan and Cribb[61]). Health promotion specialists dispense their skills and services only to those people who voluntarily seek their assistance. Leaving aside the question of whether mass public campaigns truly obtain individual informed consent (How is consent secured, for example, in large-scale social marketing campaigns?), the more troubling issue is why the field wants to develop technologies that are liable to misuse in the first place? If the potential for coercion is a problem, why do we persist in going down this path? Given the nature of contemporary threats to health, wouldn't it be better to develop ethically unproblematic (or even more strongly, ethically commendable) practices from the outset to guide and inform all our interactions with individuals and community groups? As we look toward the future, mounting financial pressures promise to put further strains on the already thin line between voluntary consent and coercive measures to force people to adopt certain behaviors.

But I have another, deeper concern. The issue involves the relationship between means and ends. When one thinks about the world in instrumental terms, means and ends tend to be viewed as independent of one another in the following sense. One can define and characterize the goal independently of the means used to achieve it. Weight loss, for example, can be defined and measured regardless of whether the means used to achieve it are a sensible diet and exercise, diet pills, liposuction, or colon staples. From an instrumental perspective, different means are regarded as interchangeable techniques, and barring side effects, the outcomes are considered independent of the means used to produce them. (I do not mean to suggest that everyone now sees these different means as equivalent, but I do think that, with the increasing resort to cost–benefit calculations, it is becoming increasingly difficult for all of us to articulate and appreciate their underlying ethical differences.) Since the results are not defined in terms of the methods, the most important question from an instrumental perspective, and the one that is currently absorbing the preponderance of the field's resources, is determining which means are most effective.

But when one is concerned with normative questions in the social world, ends cannot be characterized independently of the means. For instance, one can achieve honesty only by acting honestly. Likewise, one becomes courageous by doing courageous deeds. This book argues that well-being is just such a normative value, where means and ends are inseparable. Conceptually, this book introduces a framework of "virtues" to move away from the separate, independent, means–ends rationality characteristic of current thinking in the field and to indicate the inextricable relationship between means and ends in social life. The product is defined, at least in part, through the process by which it is achieved. In the concept of virtue, we will see that something can be both a cause and a constituent element of the ends being sought.[62]

The sociologist Robert Bellah spells out the implications for health promotion:

> The purpose . . . is not to produce or control anything but to discover through mutual discussion and reflection between free citizens the most appropriate ways, under present conditions, of living the ethically good life. . . . It is precisely the point about *praxis* [social practice] that it has no extraneous product. It has an end, namely, the good of human beings, but that end is attained through itself, that is, through action or practice that is ethical and political. . . . For 'helping professionals,' this would involve toleration of high levels of uncertainty in trying to aid people to improve their own skills of practical autonomy, rather than categorizing them in terms of preconceived theories with resulting automatic formulas for treatment.[63]

The different ways of thinking about health and well-being—instrumentally versus practically—lie at the bottom of nagging intuitions that there are important differences in terms of the quality of outcomes depending on how we get there. It does make a difference, for example, whether young people consciously and deliberately choose not to use drugs, or whether their attitudes are effectively altered through "indirect influence techniques" and "conditioning in low thought situations." Likewise, people may lose weight by taking pills, but they will not gain the dignity and self-respect that comes through exercising self-control. As the field heads down the path of technical efficiency, we are in danger of losing sight of how different means affect the quality of outcomes. To promote well-being, the means must be consonant with the ends to be achieved. We cannot promote integrity, autonomy, responsibility, caring, trust, or justice through the exercise of power—through the development of more effective techniques—no matter how strictly protocols for obtaining voluntary consent are enforced.

Fortunately, there is a tradition in health education that has worked to strengthen individual autonomy and social solidarity through practices centered on caring and fulfilling our collective responsibility for creating more humane living conditions for all people. Change and growth are possible when community members connect with one another as human beings in caring relationships characterized by trust and mutual support. It is a type of health promotion practice that is fully accountable, yet not dependent on exercising instrumental power to accomplish predetermined outcome objectives. It is based on the knowledge that, with a modicum of trust and institutional support, many good things can happen—many we may never have even considered before listening to, learning from, and engaging with fellow community members. This book is written on behalf of this group of dissenters, to justify the merits of an alternative approach and to articulate more fully the basis of our conviction that this work is good work, even if it will never meet the standards of randomized control trials. *An Ethic for Health Promotion* lays the foundation for a sound, cogent, and urgently needed alternative philosophy and practice to succeed the quest for a science of health promotion.

2

CONTEMPORARY THREATS TO HEALTH

Holyoke, Massachusetts embodies all the challenges and possibilities facing the field of health promotion. The town provides a point of reference, a reality test for the ideas developed in the chapters that follow. In Holyoke, I try to show how seemingly arcane philosophical issues have concrete, tangible repercussions that affect day-to-day activities in this field.

Holyoke is a town of 43,000 people located in semirural western Massachusetts, about 10 miles south of the University of Massachusetts, Amherst. In its inception, it was a planned city, with a bustling gridwork of canals to power the once great New England paper mills. The mills are now closed, and like many small, declining industrial towns across the Northeast, the city faces an uncertain future. Life is hard in Holyoke, although perhaps not as hard as in many large urban centers.

At the time of the 1990 census, about one-third of the population was Puerto Rican. The Puerto Rican presence is a relatively new feature in Holyoke, the result of a vast influx of migrant labor to the area over the past 2 decades. Their share of the population continues to grow. More than half of the Latinos living in Holyoke are under the age of 19.[1]

The overall age-adjusted mortality rate in Holyoke is 50% higher than in the rest of the state (659.6/100,000 versus 463.6). About 300 people die here each year. If living conditions were the same as in other communities, only 200 people would pass away. The top 10 leading causes of death in Holyoke appear in the same order as in the rest of Massachusetts and the nation—heart disease, cancer, strokes, etc.—but each is about 50% higher, with the exception of homicide, which is four times higher.[2]

In 1994, Holyoke had the highest teen pregnancy rate in Massachusetts, the second highest infant mortality rate, and the highest rate of women receiving inadequate prenatal care. The rate of teen births is four times higher than the rest of the state. Holyoke has the highest rate of domestic violence and the second highest rate of child abuse in Massachusetts.

Between 1988 and 1992, the number of confirmed AIDS cases in Holyoke went up by 500%. Holyoke AIDS rates are four times as high as state rates. Even though Latinos compose only one-third of the population, 75% of the AIDS cases are Latino. The AIDS rate among Holyoke women is twice the state average. The primary mode of transmission of AIDS in Holyoke is injection drug use, fully 63% of current cases compared to 35% statewide. The rates of different sexually transmitted diseases—syphilis, gonorrhea, chlamydia—are 300%, 30%, and 46% higher, respectively, in Holyoke than in Massachusetts as a whole. Residents here get admitted to drug treatment programs at about three times the state's rate.

According to the United States Census Bureau, the unemployment rate in 1990 in Holyoke was 10.1%, compared to 6.9% for all of Massachusetts. The unemployment rate among Holyoke Latinos was 27.1%. The average per capita income in Massachusetts that year was $17,224; in Holyoke as a whole, $11,088; among Latinos in Holyoke, $4,131. The poverty rate in Massachusetts was 11.3%, in Holyoke as a whole, 25.7%, and among Holyoke Latinos, 59.1%, for Latino children (under 12 years of age), 71.4%. Among Latino female-headed households in Holyoke, the poverty rate in 1990 was a stunning 93.1%.

The town of Holyoke captures many of the complex challenges public health must now confront. There are glaring disparities in health that cry out for relief. The problems are compounded, with drugs and AIDS and violence not falling into discrete categories but linked in individual lives. The problems are exacerbated by poverty, inequality, and racial animosities. Reflecting the concerns of the NIH panel raised in the first chapter, the School Board has banned sex education in the schools and the City Council has rejected the introduction of a needle exchange program. The community is deeply divided over these issues.

Public health professionals work at the city health department, at a federally funded community health center, at a local nonprofit hospital, in the schools, and in several small community-based organizations, such as the Care Center and Nueva Esperanza, that provide a variety of health and human services. Many of these women and men grew up here and still live in the city. As they look out of their offices, while the problems are complex, the numbers are not overwhelming: 9 infant mortality deaths, 44 new AIDS cases, 96 births to teens under 18 years of age, and 7 homicides last year. These are numbers on a human scale, not anonymous masses. As someone who is responsible for training public health professionals, I constantly ask myself, what are the people who work in these agencies in Holyoke supposed to do?

How should we think about promoting individual and community well-being in Holyoke? Should we approach these questions as fundamentally technical problems of reducing and eliminating risky behaviors, just like the health department now eliminates contaminants in the water supply? Is this what I am supposed to be training public health professionals to do? Will science discover the answers that will enable health promoters working in Holyoke to achieve public health goals? If not science, where else do we have to turn? Let us take a look at how the field's thinking about these issues has evolved over time.

A SHORT HISTORY OF HEALTH PROMOTION

The targets of health promotion and disease prevention efforts have changed over time. One schema for charting these shifts is the public health model. It is the customary foundation used in epidemiology for explaining patterns of disease.[3]

According to the public health model, health and disease are the product of the interaction of three key elements: the agent, host, and environment. Agent refers to the necessary etiologic factors, such as bacteria, chemicals, or nutritive elements (e.g., cholesterol). Host refers to the human body and its intrinsic susceptibility, exposure, and response to etiologic agents. The environment refers to extrinsic influences, including the physical, biologic, and socioeconomic environments. To explain the distribution of disease in human populations, the public health model examines the interaction and relative importance of these three elements.

From ancient times down through the modern era, the prime target of public health interventions has been the physical environment.[4] These efforts revolve around things like building sewage systems, securing a safe water supply, and draining swamps. The early focus on the physical environment grew out of Hippocrates's classic exposition, *Airs, Waters, and Places*.

In a text that would guide people's thinking about health for well over 2000 years, Hippocrates described his approach to understanding health conditions:

> Whoever wishes to investigate medicine properly should proceed thus: in the first place to consider the seasons of the year, and what effects each of them produces (for they are not all alike, but differ much from themselves in regard to their changes). Then the winds, the hot and the cold, especially such as are common to all countries, and then such as are peculiar to each locality. We must also consider the qualities of the waters, for as they differ from one another in taste and weight, so also do they differ much in their qualities. In the same manner, when one comes into a city to which he is a stranger, he ought to consider its situation, how it lies to the winds and the rising of the sun; for its influence is not the same whether it lies to the north or

the south, to the rising or the setting sun. These things one ought to consider most attentively.[5]

Dating from 400 B.C., this framework governed thinking about health for more than 23 centuries.

The rise of modern science challenged and eventually overthrew ancient Hippocratic explanations. As scientists became more successful in identifying the causes of disease, a shift of attention occurred in public health toward the end of the nineteenth century. Based on the pioneering work of Koch, Pasteur, Jenner, and others, there was an explosion of scientific discoveries—all within a short 20-year span between 1880 and 1900—of virtually all known infectious disease-causing bacteria, including typhoid, malaria, leprosy, tuberculosis, streptococcus, cholera, diphtheria, staphylococcus, tetanus, pneumococcus, and the plague.[6] Adopting and extending the new methods of scientific research, Koch's Postulates defined the procedures for determining the necessary and sufficient causes of disease.

Koch's Postulates specify four criteria: the organism is always present when the disease is present; the disease is not present in the absence of the organism; the introduction of the organism produces the disease in experimental animals; and the introduction of the organism in experimental animals does not produce other diseases.[7] Using these criteria, scientists identified the etiologic agents responsible for the leading causes of death at the turn of the century. With this wave of discoveries, attention in public health shifted to the role of the agent in the genesis of disease. This shift, from the environment to the agent, is sometimes referred to as the "first revolution" in public health.[8] With the discovery and development of immunizations, pasteurization, sterilization, antiseptic technique, and later antibiotics, scientists produced powerful new technologies for preventing and treating infectious diseases.

There is some dispute these days about whether the ensuing decline in infectious diseases should be attributed to the distribution of vaccines and antibiotics or to the rising standard of living brought about by the Industrial Revolution.[9] McKinlay and McKinlay present compelling evidence that the decline in infectious diseases began long before the discovery and development of these new weapons in the public health arsenal and they attribute the decrease primarily to improved material conditions.[10] In any case, whether through killing bacteria or cleaning up the environment, sometime between 1920 and 1940, influenza, pneumonia, and tuberculosis fell from being the leading causes of death in the United States.[11] As infectious diseases declined, they were eclipsed by new health problems—heart disease, cancer, and strokes. In time, these would come to be called chronic "lifestyle" diseases.

The etiology of chronic diseases was initially puzzling to researchers. As the Surgeon General (1979) would later remark, "During the 1950s and 1960s, a lack of knowledge about their causes led to a decline in emphasis on prevention."[12] Based on the procedures defined by Koch's Postulates, scientists continued to search for bacterial agents as the underlying basis for cancer and heart disease until well into the 1960s. They wanted to find the germ that caused cancer, and then, heading down a well-worn path, develop a vaccine, antibiotic, or other procedure that could quell its virulence. This line of research did not prove successful.

As researchers grew frustrated in their search for the microbes responsible for the development of cancer and heart disease, a new set of public health studies laid the groundwork for a major reformulation in thinking about the causes of chronic diseases. The landmark Framingham heart disease study began in the early 1950s. Set in a small town in Massachusetts, the Framingham study is now one of the best known studies in public health history. Using a prospective, longitudinal research design, Drs. Dawber, Kannell, and others collected information on a plethora of clinical, behavioral, and demographic measures from a group of 6507 males between the ages of 30 and 60 years.[13] The health status of these men was closely monitored over time, as researchers looked for commonalities among those suffering heart attacks. The results of this study are now part of the stock of common knowledge: the major causes of heart disease are smoking, cholesterol, and hypertension.

The Framingham study is significant for two reasons. First, the Framingham researchers found that the causes of chronic diseases differed in several respects from the causes of infectious diseases. The agents were chemical (e.g., cholesterol), not biological; hence, they could not be controlled through immunizations, pasteurization, antibiotics, or other known technologies. Moreover, these agents of disease did not share the same necessary and sufficient causal relationship found between bacteria and infectious diseases.

To explain the causes of chronic diseases, epidemiologists had to redefine causality in terms of probabilities. As the analysis of the data dictated, the agents of chronic disease were redefined as "risk factors." A particular risk factor was neither a necessary nor sufficient cause of a specific disease; it was seen only to make the onset of a given chronic disease more likely. It is from the Framingham study and other similar investigations that the concept of probabilistic risk factors gained its place in the public health lexicon of disease processes.

The Framingham study was also important in instigating the "second revolution" in public health.[14] Its results led to a growing recognition of the crucial role human behaviors play in the etiology of chronic diseases. A convenient marker for dating the start of the second revolution in public health is the release of the United States Surgeon General's *Report on Smoking and Health* in 1964, which documented the health consequences of smoking on cancer, heart disease, and other major illnesses. As the impact of human behaviors in chronic disease processes came to be more fully appreciated, the center of public health attention shifted once again, this time from the agent to the host.

Across the country, the results of another well-known study, started in 1964 at the Human Population Laboratory (HPL) in Alameda County, California, added to the growing weight of evidence demonstrating the impact of host behaviors on the leading causes of morbidity and mortality. At the HPL, Nedra Belloc and Lester Breslow found that seven health habits were consistently associated with higher rates of heart attacks: (1) cigarette smoking, (2) weight to height ratio, (3) the number of hours of sleep each night, (4) whether or not one eats breakfast, (5) whether one eats snacks between meals, (6) level of physical activity, and (7) the amount of alcohol consumption.[15] Additional studies based on the HPL data are also significant for calling attention to the role of the sociocultural environment in the etiology of modern chronic diseases.

The first major reanalysis of the HPL data was conducted by an epidemiologist named Lisa Berkman.[16] Using crude indicators, Berkman discovered that social involvement and social support have a major impact on people's health, near or equal in magnitude to the previously studied individual health habits. The crude measure of social support that Berkman used had only four items: (1) whether married or not; (2) whether attends church regularly or not; (3) whether member of a social club or not; and, (4) whether visits with friends regularly or not. But even with this rudimentary scale, Berkman found a robust relationship between social support and the likelihood of suffering a heart attack. The more socially engaged people are, the less likely they will suffer ill-health, and conversely, the more isolated, the greater the threat to their health. Berkman demonstrated that the relationship holds up even after statistically controlling for the effects of various health behaviors.

Along about the same time, a number of studies started coming out in the mid-to late 1960s that documented the impact of poverty and social class on health. The first major review of these data was conducted by Anton Antonovsky. Leonard Syme summarizes his findings: "In a comprehensive review of over 30 studies, Antonovsky concluded that those in the lower classes invariably have lower life expectancy and higher death rates from all causes of death, and that this higher rate has been observed since the twelfth century when data on this question were first organized."[17]

Because of the way data are collected and analyzed, the effects of social class on health have been more extensively studied in Great Britain than in the United States. Data there are collected using the British Registrar-General's classification scheme that delineates six social classes: professionals; employers and managers; skilled (nonmanual) occupations; skilled manual labor; semiskilled and personal services; and, nonskilled manual labor. Using this measure of social class, Michael Marmot and his colleagues have found a remarkably consistent relationship between socioeconomic status and disease.[18] Across a broad range of indicators, from birthweight to infant mortality, childhood mortality, maternal mortality, coronary heart disease, and respiratory diseases to measures of morbidity like the average number of restricted activity days and bouts of chronic illnesses to measures of risk factors like smoking and the lack of exercise, there is a steady and robust gradient with stepwise declines in health at each descending level of socioeconomic status (SES). Across virtually all indicators, health is consistently worse the lower the social class.

In the United States, the relative impact of income, social support, and lifestyle behaviors on health was then examined by Mary Haan and her colleagues, using the same data collected by Belloc and Breslow at the Human Population Laboratory.[19] Haan, et al., reanalyzed the available information to investigate the relationship between income and health, comparing residents living in federally designated poverty areas with those living in nonpoverty neighborhoods. Even with this rather crude measure, they found that, to take but one example, the mortality rate for white males aged 35–44 was 12.5 per 1000 among those living in poverty areas versus 3.9 per 1000 for nonpoverty residents.[20] They then looked at the impact of SES relative to the health habits identified by Belloc and Breslow in earlier studies (smoking, alcohol consumption, body mass, etc.).

Epidemiologists have developed a measure, called relative risk, to gauge the effect of exposure to suspected risk factors. In relative risk calculations, the death rates of those with a particular risk factor are compared to the rates of those who do not have it. Haan and her colleagues found that the relative risk for premature death due to health habits was 1.54. People who smoke, drink, are overweight, do not exercise, and so on, are 1.54 times more likely to die in a given year than people who do not smoke, do not drink, get regular exercise, are not overweight, etc. Turning to income, the relative risk for people living in poverty areas when compared to those living in nonpoverty areas was 1.50, after controlling for the influence of health habits. When race is added to the measure of socioeconomic status, the relative risk jumps to 1.71. For social support, the relative risk for heart disease due to social isolation was 1.47.[21] In sum, the results of Haan's study show that SES has a comparable, if not greater, and independent impact on people's health over and above their individual health habits. The strength of the relationship is approximately equal to that of social support too, again after controlling for their independent contributions.

The Framingham study, the *Surgeon General's Report on Smoking and Health*, the various HPL studies, and the studies by Antonovsky and Marmot laid the foundation for a series of major reports that have defined priorities for the field of health promotion through the end of the millennium. The two major streams of findings—those looking at individual behaviors and those looking at socioeconomic and sociocultural influences—culminated in a pair of reports that capture current thinking about health promotion.

In 1974, Marc LaLonde, then Minister of Health Services in Canada, released *A New Perspective on the Health of Canadians*. The report is momentous because it was the first major national planning document to declare that behavioral factors, or "unhealthy lifestyles," are the most important determinant of health status in modern times. The other three major categorical influences identified in the LaLonde report are environmental factors (including economic), biological (genetic) factors, and medical care.[22]

Shortly thereafter, the United States Surgeon General commissioned and published *Healthy People: The Surgeon General's Report On Health Promotion and Disease Prevention.* Issued in 1979, this report defined the health goals for America for the decade ending in 1990. Following the lead of the groundbreaking LaLonde report, *Healthy People* cited the increasing significance of health behaviors, but then went one step beyond the Canadian document. *Healthy People* attached a quantitative estimate of the relative significance of each of the four categories identified by LaLonde. According to the United States Surgeon General, "Using that [*New Perspective*] framework, a group of American experts developed a method for assessing the relative contributions of each of the elements to many health problems. Analysis in which the method was applied to the 10 leading causes of death in 1976 suggests that perhaps as much as half of mortality in 1976 in the United States was due to unhealthy behavior or lifestyle; 20% to environmental factors; 20% to human biological factors; and only 10% to inadequacies in health care."[23] So stated, *Healthy People* declared that half of all deaths in the United States were attributable to individual behaviors.

Finally, in a parallel effort that came to a different conclusion, the Department of Health and Social Security (DHSS) commissioned a national public health planning document for Great Britain in 1976. The Commission was headed by Sir Douglas Black, then president of the Royal College of Physicians. Their final document is commonly referred to as the Black Report.[24]

Based on the findings reported by Marmot and others, the British Health Commission systematically examined four rival hypotheses regarding the observed relationship between social class and health status: (*1*) the observed differences were an artifact of statistical analyses; (*2*) the differences were due to "natural selection," i.e., poor health leads to a lower income, rather than the other way round; (*3*) the "cultural explanation"—social classes differentially socialize people into behaviors and customs related to health like diet, smoking, alcohol, exercise, and so on; and, (*4*) the "materialist explanation"—health differences are due to differences in material conditions. After methodically ruling out the first three explanations, the Black Commission came to the conclusion that the distribution of health problems in Great Britain was primarily due to economic inequalities. The Black report, officially entitled *Inequalities in Health*, concluded that a major redistribution in wealth would be necessary to effect improvements in the overall health status of people in Great Britain.

One full century after the first, the second revolution in public health is thus marked by this shift in attention and concern. The onus of responsibility for the leading causes of death has been relocated, displaced from infectious agents and the physical environment to individual host behaviors and the social environment. Due to the history of its previous successes, where dramatic reductions in disease prevalence were achieved through cleaning up an unsanitary physical environment and immobilizing the agents of infectious disease, the field of public health promotion is now applying these same thought patterns to modern health problems. Since the start of the second revolution in public health about 30 years ago, research priorities have been set and resources have been mobilized in order to achieve comparable control over contemporary threats to health. But, where in an earlier era, the field targeted pathogens borne by an unsanitary physical environment, now we are targeting volitions borne by a troubled sociocultural environment.

PROGRESS THROUGH SCIENCE

For those committed to the development of a science of health promotion, progress will be achieved through testing and proving scientific theories regarding human behavior. These theories provide the basis for developing more effective behavioral interventions. Specifically, the aim of health promotion research is to advance explanatory theories that identify the risk factors that cause (or, in probabilistic terms, make more likely) those behaviors that compromise health. Once identified, the logic of this approach dictates that reducing or eliminating those risk factors will result in changes in behavior, which in turn will lead to lower morbidity and mortality rates.

Two points follow from the commitment to the scientific method. First, the research designs that are used to study human behavior are no different than the research designs used to examine biological processes. Under the prevailing system of grant-funded research, the process of developing and testing theories of behavior is exactly the same as the experimental, hypothesis-testing procedures used in the biomedical sciences.

Second, the conduct of scientific research prescribes the design of health promotion programs. The strongest type of evidence establishing cause-and-effect relationships in scientific research—that which allows researchers to say with certainty that a suspected risk factor is definitely to blame—comes from conducting experiments. In experimental research, a suspected risk factor must be modified—increased or decreased—in order to observe the effect of this variation on the dependent variable. Thus, the techniques that researchers use to test hypotheses about the effect of antecedent risk factors on consequent behaviors, when successful, become the techniques that practitioners should use to effect changes in health-related behaviors. Because of this congruence, it is important to begin with a clear picture of the research process and the relationship between theory and practice in the conventional view.

The process of identifying and verifying risk factors goes through a sequence of stages. These stages have been formally codified in protocols developed by the National Cancer Institute of the National Institutes of Health.[25] (See Figure 2–1.) Stage I involves Hypothesis Development, basic exploratory research at the most rudimentary level. Research at this stage is a broad open-ended search for any potential factors that might possibly play a role in the etiology of the health problem under investigation. Stage I research may be "qualitative" in the sense that the research designs are not required to measure or count things rigorously at this stage.

Stage II research centers on Methods Development. Based on findings from Stage I, once investigators suspect a particular factor is involved, they then set out to measure it systematically and observe whether it fluctuates consistently with the problem of interest. Where there is more of one, is there more of the other? and vice versa. More cholesterol, more heart disease, for instance. In Stage II, researchers develop "operational definitions": detailed descriptions of the instruments used to measure the objects under investigation. Operational definitions allow everyone to know exactly how the suspected risk factor and outcomes were measured. They are objective indicators, which enable others to replicate the study.

If significant correlations are found in Stage II, the research moves to Stage III, Controlled Intervention Trials. In Stage III research, the investigators test hypotheses about the relationship between the specific risk factor and outcome of interest. Stage III research entails discrete, independent, small scale, often laboratory tests of hypotheses. Going one step beyond correlations, hypothesis-testing establishes the chronological relationship between cause and effect.

Stage IV research, Defined Population Studies, involves large-scale, coordinated tests involving multiple sites, to confirm the generalizability of the results. In the recent COMMIT trials, for example, the National Cancer Institute selected 22 cities for testing hypotheses about whether smoking prevalence could be reduced through interventions targeting selected risk factors. Finally, at Stage V, Demonstration and Implementation, the results of successful interventions are disseminated on a national level.

In similar fashion, researchers have developed a system for grading the caliber of research results. Based on rules of evidence, studies are assigned to a five-level ranking system indicative of the confidence attached to the findings. Randomized control trials with low false positive (alpha) and low false negative (beta) errors are rated at Level I; randomized control trials with high false positive or high false negative errors are rated Level II; nonrandomized cohort studies are rated Level III; and nonrandomized historical cohort studies and case studies receive the lowest rankings, Levels IV and V, respectively.[26]

Under these protocols, all health research lies on a road that culminates in large scale experimental tests of hypotheses. Anything less merits less confidence and

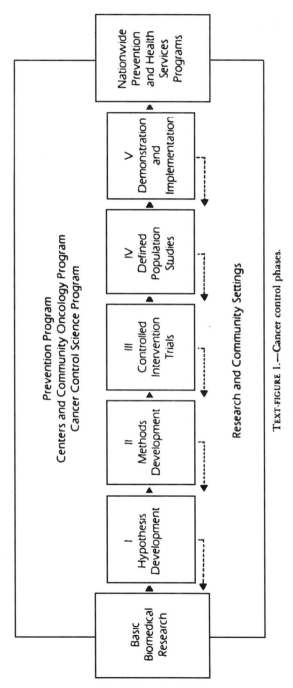

Prevention Program
Centers and Community Oncology Program
Cancer Control Science Program

Basic Biomedical Research	I Hypothesis Development	II Methods Development	III Controlled Intervention Trials	IV Defined Population Studies	V Demonstration and Implementation	Nationwide Prevention and Health Services Programs

Research and Community Settings

TEXT-FIGURE 1.—Cancer control phases.

FIGURE 2–1. Stages of research. Used with permission, Greenwald, et al. (1987).

a lower ranking. Interventions that have not been tested following these protocols are not considered satisfactory for dissemination. After proving the efficacy of the intervention under investigation, the results are then disseminated nationally. This research framework prescribes the practice of health promotion.

In experimental research, researchers formulate hypotheses about relationships between cause and effect. Hypotheses are predictions using an "If–Then" formula: If X happens, then Y will happen, If X goes up, then Y will go up. Researchers might hypothesize, for instance, about the relationship between self-esteem and teenage drug use. A typical hypothesis might be that low self-esteem causes, or makes more likely, the onset of youthful drug abuse. Researchers then test hypotheses by predicting the changes in the dependent variable that will occur as a result of changes in the independent variable(s). In the standard formula: If low self-esteem is reduced, then drug use will go down.

To test hypotheses (Stages III and IV), researchers begin by randomly assigning subjects to "treatment" and "control" groups. Random assignment is used to insure that the people in each group are alike, thus minimizing the possibility that any extraneous, unintended differences between the two groups might bias the results of the experiment. In studies of teenage drug abuse, individual students, classrooms, or even whole schools are routinely randomly assigned to treatment or control conditions.

The investigators then conduct the experiment: they implement an intervention in the treatment group. In health promotion research, interventions are designed to alter hypothesized risk factors. The treatment group might receive medications intended to control their blood pressure, nicotine patches to suppress the urge to smoke, social inoculations to resist peer pressure, or positive reinforcements to boost their self-esteem. Researchers then measure whether the intervention modifies the targeted risk factor as intended, and consequently, whether lower disease incidence rates result over time. Statistical tests are used to certify the significance of the effects by estimating the probability that any observed differences are due to chance. Such Randomized Control Trials (RCTs) are the gold standard of NIH research.

Under these protocols, the procedures used to test hypotheses about behavioral influences are identical to those used to test hypotheses about physiological processes. Support from the NIH culminates in Randomized Control Trials, whether for trials of new medications for treating AIDS or for testing school-based drug abuse prevention curricula. Experimental research is the ideal against which all other research is measured. Decisions about which research receives funding are based largely on the degree to which researchers can approximate ideal experimental conditions or show that the proposed research is an essential preliminary step in the sequence of stages leading toward fully experimental tests of hypotheses.

There is one further major implication for the practice of health promotion that follows from this commitment to the development of a science of health promotion. Based on these methods of research, the development of interventions is inherent in the process of testing theories and hypotheses. An alleged gap between theory and practice is frequently lamented at health promotion conferences. There are good reasons for the breakdown between theory and practice as they are currently construed, reasons which we discuss in the next chapter. But for now, it is important to see the congruence between theory and practice established by the model of experimental research. Based on this model, there should be no gap—the techniques used in research to test the effects of the independent variable on the dependent variable are the techniques that can, will, and should be used in practice. Based on the results of successful experiments, practitioners learn exactly what they are supposed to do to effect change. Clinicians learn which medications are effective and which are not. Likewise, health promotion specialists learn which techniques are effective in changing antecedent risk factors and which are effective in changing behaviors. As Glanz, Lewis, and Rimer note, "researchers must do precisely what practitioners do—develop and deliver interventions."[27]

To illustrate the isomorphic relationship between research and practice in the scientific model, let us take a closer look at the relationship as it now functions in the field.[28] Following the above procedures, health promotion researchers have developed and tested a relatively well-defined set of theories. The names of these theories are familiar to anyone in the field: the Health Belief Model, Social Learning Theory, the Theory of Reasoned Action, the Diffusion of Innovations, Cognitive Dissonance Theory, the Theory of Protection Motivation, the Transtheoretical Model, Social Marketing, Social Support Theory, and so on.[29] Each of these theories has identified a small number of discrete independent variables (typically 4–6) that have been shown to cause or make more likely change in the dependent variable, i.e., people's behavior. To use the Health Belief Model as an example, researchers have repeatedly demonstrated that increasing people's "perceived susceptibility" (their perception of the likelihood they will contract a given disease) results in behavior change: taking action to decrease their susceptibility.

Theories that have demonstrated the power to effect change have been grouped into four major categories: (*1*) Behaviorist—the use of positive and negative reinforcements (e.g., punishing teenagers who smoke at school, contests that reward employees who lose the most weight); (*2*) Persuasive Communications—the use of fear appeals, one-sided versus two-sided arguments, sex appeals, subliminal messages, etc.; (*3*) Group Pressure—placement in reference groups to gain compliance with identified norms (e.g., court referrals to Alcoholics Anonymous); and, (*4*) Direct Instrumental Power—the use of positions of authority (e.g., doctor's orders), public policy (e.g., banning smoking, mandating seat belt use), and mass mobilizations (e.g., demonstrations, sit-ins, etc.).[30]

Health promotion specialists are taught these theories in academic training programs. Through courses on theory, program planning, and evaluation, the process of putting theory into practice is made explicit.

To apply theory, the prevailing view directs the practitioner to start by conducting a baseline "needs assessment" of the independent variables specified in a given theory. The baseline survey is used to determine the most effective targets for intervention. To put the Health Belief Model into practice in preventing AIDS, the practitioner should conduct a preintervention survey of the model's six independent variables: perceived susceptibility to AIDS, perceived severity of AIDS, perceived barriers to changing behavior, perceived benefits to changing behavior, cues to action (socioenvironmental prompts, such as a doctor's advice), and, with its recent incorporation into the model, perceived self-efficacy. From this baseline survey of the target population, the practitioner gains information about the most strategic sites for effecting change. For example, she might learn that the perceptions of the severity of AIDS in a given population are high, but their perceived susceptibility to AIDS and perceived self-efficacy in using condoms (or cleaning needles) are low. From this information, she then knows that interventions for this population need not focus on increasing their perception of the severity of AIDS (since it is already high), but instead would achieve better results by concentrating on increasing their perceived susceptibility and self-efficacy.[31]

After completing the needs assessment, the practitioner needs to decide which interventions to carry out in order to increase or decrease those strategically salient variables identified in the baseline survey. Here is how theory and research inform the choice of interventions. To increase perceived susceptibility, the practitioner needs to persuade listeners that they are likely to get the disease. She could start by citing statistics about disease prevalence rates for the target population. But from other information dissemination theories, such as the Diffusion of Innovations, she would know that it is more effective to invite a speaker who has many characteristics in common with the target audience and is HIV+. In tests of the Diffusion of Innovations Theory, researchers have shown that *homophilous* sources—people who share many characteristics in common with the target audience—are more effective in producing changes in beliefs than people who are unlike [*heterophilous*] the target audience. To increase perceived self-efficacy (i.e., confidence in their ability to carry out the recommended behavior), she should demonstrate how to use a condom and ask the audience to practice the behavior. These interventions are borrowed from Social Learning Theory where the concept of self-efficacy was first developed. In tests of Social Learning Theory, researchers have demonstrated the effectiveness of *modeling* and *behavioral rehearsal* in effecting behavior change.

To evaluate the program, practitioners are urged to conduct follow-up surveys. (In research designs, these are called "post-tests." Follow-up evaluation surveys yield the same information that researchers collect after conducting experiments, although practitioners may forego the use of a control group, depending on the situation.) From a follow-up survey, a practitioner can learn many things. First, she can find out if the intervention had its intended impact: did the target audience's perceived susceptibility and perceived self-efficacy increase compared to the level at the time of the baseline survey? Since the effects of homophily, modeling, and behavioral rehearsal have already been proven, ineffective programs are presumed to be the result of a breakdown or attenuation in the fidelity of applying these constructs. If the follow-up survey indicates no effect, the practitioner is advised to double check whether implementation was consistent with the operational definitions used in the research, e.g., did the students actually rehearse using a condom (whereby their self-efficacy would be increased)?

Second, she may learn something about the magnitude of change. Common measures of constructs like perceived susceptibility and perceived self-efficacy are five-point scales, running from (1)—"Not at all" susceptible or confident to (5)—"Highly" susceptible or confident. A program that causes a three-point shift in people's perceptions (say, from an average of 1.5 at the time of baseline to 4.5 after the intervention) is considered more effective, and hence more likely to effect behavior change, than a program that causes a half-point shift. This information is usually most helpful to practitioners in advocating for additional resources. She can demonstrate that a 2-week program is insufficient to effect change and that an 8-week program is more effective than a 4-week program. (Researchers term this phenomenon "dose response," the effect is proportional to the amount of the intervention.)

Finally, she will learn if the changes in the identified variables produce the desired changes in behavior. At baseline and follow-up, she can ask the target audience how frequently they use condoms. If condom use has gone up as predicted by increases in perceived susceptibility and self-efficacy, then the program is considered a success. Effecting behavior change is ultimately the whole point of utilizing social and behavioral theories. It is the science of health promotion.

HEALTHY PEOPLE

The results of the various research programs sponsored by the NIH and other agencies feed directly into federal public health planning documents. *Healthy People* was originally released in 1979. Its sequel, *Healthy People 2000*, was published in 1990 and it details the goals and objectives for public health promotion in the United States through the year 2000. These reports are the principal planning documents that set forth the basic framework and strategies now envisioned for promoting the nation's health.

As head of the United States Public Health Service, the Surgeon General's plan guides the activities of all agencies that fall under its jurisdiction: the Centers for Disease Control, the Food and Drug Administration, the Health Resources and Services Administration, the Agency for Toxic Substances and Disease Registry, the Substance Abuse and Mental Health Administration, and the National Institutes of Health. As a gross indicator of the scope and influence of these organizations, the combined resources of the United States Public Health Service in 1996 amounted to $23.25 billion in expenditures. The research and programs sponsored by these agencies set the agenda for local public health promotion efforts.

The original *Healthy People* report in 1979 specified five goals for the nation to be accomplished by 1990:

- to reduce infant mortality by at least 35%;
- to reduce deaths among children ages 1–14 by at least 20%;
- to reduce deaths among people ages 15–24 by at least 20 percent;
- to reduce deaths among people ages 25–64 by at least 25%; and,
- to reduce the average annual number of days of restricted activity due to acute and chronic conditions by 20%, to fewer than 30 days per year, for people aged 65 and older.

Based on these goals, the Surgeon General issued a follow-up report, *Objectives for the Nation*, in 1980. *Objectives for the Nation* spelled out the first detailed plan for promoting health on a national level. Objectives were grouped into three broad arenas: prevention, promotion, and protection. The three areas roughly correspond to the three elements in the classic public health model: agent, host, and environment, respectively. Under each area, five categorical, content-specific topics were identified for priority attention. (See Table 2–1.)

Prevention efforts focus on the control of disease-causing agents, including topics such as immunizations and sexually transmitted diseases. Protection corresponds to the environment, setting standards for the regulation of known pollutants—toxins, radiation, and other environmental hazards. Health Promotion is associated with the role of the host and individual lifestyle behaviors. The five topics in this area are smoking, the misuse of alcohol and other drugs, nutrition, physical fitness and exercise, and violence.

Using this framework, *Healthy People* specified a grand total of 226 objectives for the nation. In a progress report issued in 1990, 36 of the 226 objectives originally set in 1980 had been achieved, another 65 were on track to be achieved, 65 were unlikely to be achieved, and there were insufficient data to determine progress on the remaining 59 objectives.[32] Growing out of this experience, the Surgeon General produced a new 10-year plan, *Healthy People 2000*, in 1990. *Healthy People 2000* now guides the nation's public health promotion activities.

TABLE 2–1. Healthy People

PROMOTING HEALTH/PREVENTING DISEASE: OBJECTIVES FOR THE NATION

Preventive Health Services

High blood pressure
Family planning
Pregnancy and infant health
Immunization
Sexually transmitted diseases

Health Protection

Toxic agent control
Occupational health and safety
Accident prevention and injury control
Flouridation and dental health
Surveillance and control of infectious diseases

Health Promotion

Smoking and health
Misuse of alcohol and drugs
Nutrition
Physical fitness and exercise
Control of stress and violent behavior

Like its predecessor, *Healthy People 2000* is a blueprint for improving the health of the nation. It sets down three broad goals and 247 specific objectives for achieving a healthier society over the decade leading into the year 2000.

In response to criticisms that the goals put forward in the first *Healthy People* plan were too narrowly defined (targeted exclusively on reducing death rates), the goals of *Healthy People 2000* were modified. The three current goals for the nation are to:

- increase the span of healthy life for Americans;
- reduce health disparities among Americans; and,
- achieve access to preventive services for all Americans.

Healthy People 2000 retains its predecessor's organization of objectives into the arenas of prevention, protection, and promotion. The number of categorical topics was increased from 15 to 22 priority areas. Family planning, mental health, and educational programs have been added under Health Promotion in the new plan.

Also like its predecessor, *Healthy People 2000* organizes the objectives in each topic area into an explicit planning model that defines the logic for accomplishing the nation's goals. For each topic, there are four types of objectives: (*1*) services and protection; (2) risk reduction; (3) health status; and, (4) surveillance and data needs. The logic of this planning model was originally articulated by Dr. Lawrence Green, then head of the Office of Health Information and Health Promotion (now the Office of Disease Prevention and Health Promotion) at the time of the first *Healthy People* report.[33] Green has developed a more fully elaborated version of this planning framework, called the PRECEDE–PROCEED Model.[34]

The planning model is configured as a flow chart sequencing the relationships among the different types of objectives. (See Fig. 2–2.) The model flows like this. To achieve the nation's health goals, the first step is to improve health services. Improved health services are expected to produce increased public and professional awareness. Increased public and professional awareness will lead to risk reduction. Risk reduction in turn will result in improved health status. The final set of objectives, surveillance and data, document the impact of the intervention.

An example from the Health Promotion topic, Alcohol and Other Drugs, may serve to illustrate the model.

Under (1) Improved Services and Protection, *Healthy People 2000* states:

- "Provide to children in all school districts and private schools primary and secondary school educational programs on alcohol and other drugs, preferably as part of quality school health education."

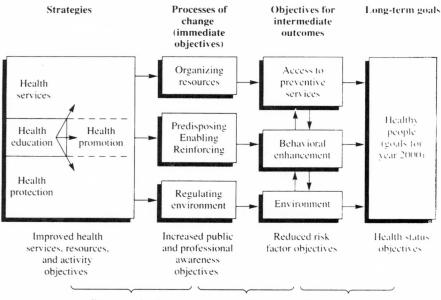

FIGURE 2–2. Health promotion planning model. Used with permission, Green and Kreuter (1991).

Under (2) Public Awareness and Risk Reduction,

- "Increase the proportion of high school seniors who associate risk of physical or psychological harm with the heavy use of alcohol, regular use of marijuana, and experimentation with cocaine."
- "Increase the proportion of high school seniors who perceive social disapproval associated with the heavy use of alcohol, occasional use of marijuana, and experimentation with cocaine."
- "Increase by at least 1 year the average age of first use of cigarettes, alcohol, and marijuana by adolescents aged 12 through 17."
- "Reduce alcohol consumption by people aged 14 and older to an annual average of no more than 2 gallons of ethanol per person."

Under (3) Improved Health Status,

- "Reduce deaths caused by alcohol-related motor vehicle crashes to no more than 8.5 per 100,000 people."

The rationales behind the two categories of objectives, Improved Health Services and Improved Health Status, are self-evident. The Risk Reduction objectives illustrate the use of behavioral science theories as they are now used in official government planning documents.

The Risk Reduction objectives contain a mix of behavioral and social–psychological risk factors. The social–psychological factors targeted are considered determinants of behavior. Building on federally funded programs of research, they are taken from well-known social scientific theories of human behavior widely used in the field. As we saw above, "Perceived Harm" is a variable identified in the Health Belief Model. "Perceived Social Norms" is a variable identified in the Theory of Reasoned Action. These variables are thought to stand in the same relation to behaviors as behaviors stand to health outcomes. They are risk factors. Just as drinking and driving makes motor vehicle crashes more likely, perceived social approval makes drinking more likely. By the same token, to reduce car crashes, we need to reduce drinking and driving, and to reduce drinking, we need to reduce social approval (or increase social disapproval). To postpone the age of first use among adolescents, their perceptions of physical and psychological harm need to be increased.

For planning purposes, the potential number of risk factors that can be targeted is unlimited.[35] In the PRECEDE model, Green classifies the "determinants of behavior" into categories he labels Predisposing, Reinforcing, and Enabling factors (hence, the PREcede model). These are generic categories into which any factors that have a demonstrated relationship to behavior change can be included. Under predisposing factors, for example, Green includes knowledge, beliefs, attitudes, values, intentions, skills, and self-efficacy, borrowing variables from at least four different social–psychological theories delineated in the research literature. McLeroy and his colleagues recommend the use of an Ecological Model.[36] The Ecological Model establishes five categories of variables: intrapersonal, interpersonal, organizational, community, and public policy. In both the PRECEDE and the Ecological Model, the identified categories provide handy heuristic labels for organizing a potentially limitless supply of variables. The PRECEDE and Ecological Models make room for the incorporation of any potential risk factor variable. Possibilities for inclusion are subject only to confirmation through scientific research.

The major research arm of the United States Public Health Service is the National Institutes of Health (NIH). The NIH house the research operations of the National Institute on Drug Abuse, the National Institute on Alcoholism and Alcohol Abuse, the National Cancer Institute, the National Institute on Aging, the National Institute of Child Health and Human Development, National Heart, Lung and Blood Institute, National Institute of Environmental Health Sciences, the National Institute of Dental Research, and the National Institute of Allergy and Infectious Diseases. The National Institutes of Health is the major source of federal support for behavioral research designed to test hypotheses about the relationship between suspected risk factors and behavioral outcomes. The NIH spent approximately $13.1 billion on health research in 1998.

PRESSURE FROM MANAGED CARE

In the early 1990s, another element entered the mix of forces shaping health promotion efforts, the rise of managed care. Managed care is the term used to capture a variety of strategies aimed at containing runaway health care costs in the United States.

As the costs of health care in the United States increased at almost twice the inflation rate throughout the 1980s (7.7% for health care versus 4.3% per annum for the Consumer Price Index), and health care costs in the United States grew at more than twice the rate of the other 24 developed countries in the world (3.2% versus 1.2%, as a percentage of the Gross Domestic Product), and the United States spent almost twice as much of its gross domestic product on health care compared to other developed countries (13.6% in the United States, compared to 8.7% in Germany and 6.9% in Japan),[37] and the United States still had a lower life expectancy and gross disparities on other indicators such as infant mortality (where the United States now ranks 24th among the world's nations), business leaders and governmental officials initiated discussions about how to control costs. In effect, the business industry has since decided to refuse to pay for increases in health insurance premiums that outpace inflation; it has thus forced the insurance industry, the hospital industry, and health care providers to figure

out how to work within limited resources.[38] Managed care means making decisions about allocating resources in order to gain maximum benefit. Insurance
companies are now deciding which procedures and which referrals they will
reimburse, and which they will not.

Health maintenance organizations (HMOs) are another form of managed care.
Enrollees pay a set premium each year for which the HMO agrees to provide all
of the health care services (covered under the contract) that one needs for the year.
The rise of managed care is a major sea change in orientation from the prior fee-
for-service system. For consumers, it matters little whether they (or more typically, their employer) pay an annual premium to an insurance company or to an
HMO, and the respective methods of finance are now converging on the types of
services they provide. Where health insurers once gave consumers great latitude
in their choice of doctor, they are now increasingly limiting those choices to doctors who are willing to work under their managed care guidelines. In 1996, approximately 85% of people with access to health care in the United States (i.e.,
not including the 44 million uninsured people in the United States) were enrolled
in some form of managed care system.[39] The rise of managed care is creating
powerful pressures on health promotion.

The most significant pressure comes from the realignment of financial incentives, leading the entire health care industry to become more invested in prevention. If providing treatment services is a drain on resources, it is in everyone's
interest to prevent people from needing them. The industry commonly refers to
health education as "demand management." So the industry is now looking to
health promotion and disease prevention specialists to deliver on their promises—
to demonstrate that they either already have or can soon develop effective techniques for preventing people from taking up behaviors that harm their health.[40]
Managed care organizations have developed their own research capacities and
research focusing on disease prevention and utilization/cost issues are among their
highest priorities.[41] The pressure to deliver demonstrably cost-effective prevention intervention techniques is growing more intense.

Currently, managed care health plans limit or deny people access to services if
the effectiveness of the services is questionable. This is most evident in mental health
care where war is being waged on a daily basis all across the country over inpatient
psychiatric hospitalizations. Insurance companies are denying payment for hospital bed days unless hospital personnel (psychiatrists or social workers) can certify
that patients pose an imminent threat to take their own or another's life. Similarly,
managed care plans are limiting the number of times a patient can enter alcohol or
drug treatment. To reduce costs, the private health care industry is aggressively reviewing services and denying those services that have not been proven to be cost-
effective. Currently, this pressure is being most intensely felt by prevention services.
Managed care is thus forcing health promotion specialists to think about their work

not as something being provided because it is a good and right thing to do, but because it is cost-effective. It saves money. It is a means to an end.

If more effective techniques are developed, there will be pressure to put them into use, thus putting increasing pressure on the relatively minimal ethical safeguards that are now in place. The industry standard is that patients must make an informed consent before undergoing any procedure. But it is obvious that doctors now possess the power to coerce patients, however subtly, because of their position of prestige and authority. If a doctor recommends a procedure, it is difficult to say no. (And these same cost-saving measures are making it increasingly difficult to get a second opinion.) Doctors now fairly routinely prescribe nicotine patches to patients who smoke, even to adolescents who may only be experimenting with cigarettes. Likewise, some corporations are now offering financial incentives to employees who maintain decent weight, blood pressure, and cholesterol levels; others, U-Haul International, for example, charge smokers and those who are more than 20% heavier than their medically ideal weight more for their health insurance.[42]

As the insurance industry and HMOs are being forced to work within fixed resources, they are also becoming more selective about whom they allow to sign up with their plans. They want to screen out people with preexisting conditions because these people will need more services, and hence, require more expenditures. This is already happening with people who smoke, people with AIDS, people with a history of mental health problems, and other health conditions. As researchers search for the antecedent social–psychological risk factors that predispose people to take up unhealthy behaviors, one wonders how long it will be before the same measures that are now used to operationalize hypothesized risk factors are used to screen out potential applicants to health care plans. Depression is a good example of where valid and reliable questionnaire scales have been developed to measure this psychological construct.

Beyond the irony of the results of health promotion research being used to deny people care, the more relevant point for my purposes is that the field of health promotion is becoming further caught up in a system of thought, a way of looking at the world, that stresses a calculative and instrumental stance toward others. The rise of managed care presses toward developing more effective and more powerful techniques for effecting changes in the way people live, with few and precarious ethical safeguards restraining their application.

THE SOCIAL ORIGINS OF MODERN MALADIES

In surveying the events shaping the field today, we have seen that, with improvements in the physical environment and the development of drugs and vaccines to combat disease-causing bacteria, the types of illnesses to which people succumb and from which they die have changed. Public and professional appreciation of these changes is relatively recent, dating roughly from the mid 1960s. This information was first used in major national public health planning documents in the late 1970s. The question raised in this book is the significance of this shift. Has our thinking about the fundamental approach to health improvement changed with the changing nature of modern ailments?

The 10 leading causes of death in the United States are listed in Table 2–2. With the exception of influenza and pneumonia (which usually stem from complications of other health problems) and AIDS, all are noninfectious diseases. Modern maladies for the most part are not caused by the invasion of microbial organisms nor from hazards in the physical environment.[43]

Table 2–2 also lists the most "prominent, controllable" risk factors associated with current health problems, as identified by Green in a widely used program

TABLE 2–2. Prominent Controllable Risk Factors for Leading Causes of Death in the United States

CAUSE OF DEATH	RISK FACTORS
Heart disease and stroke	Smoking, high blood pressure, elevated serum cholesterol, diabetes, obesity, lack of exercise
Cancer	Smoking, alcohol misuse, diet, solar radiation, ionizing radiation, worksite hazards, environmental pollution
Unintentional injuries other than motor vehicle	Alcohol misuse, smoking (fires), product design, home hazards, handgun availability
Motor vehicle injuries	Alcohol misuse, lack of safety restraints, excessive speed, automobile design, roadway design
Pneumonia and influenza	Smoking, infectious agents
Diabetes mellitus	Obesity (for adult-onset diabetes)
Cirrhosis of the liver	Alcohol ingestion
Suicide	Handgun availability, alcohol or drug misuse, stress
Homicide	Handgun availability, alcohol or drug misuse, stress
AIDS	Sexual practices, drug misuse, exposure to blood products

Used with permission, Green and Kreuter (1991).

planning text in the field today.[44] As a perusal of the list makes clear, the vast majority of contemporary threats to health arise as a consequence of human behaviors. (Even with AIDS—in many respects a throwback to an earlier era when infectious diseases were the leading causes of death—behaviors will necessarily continue to be the central focus of prevention efforts until vaccines or medications to control or kill the virus are developed.)

The list, as published, is notable in another respect. It displays an indiscriminate mixture of different types of risk factors. The list is an amalgam of items that makes no distinction between threats posed by the environment, the agent, or the host. Is there a difference? Should we think about reducing cholesterol consumption in the same way that we think about reducing environmental pollution? Does the shift in the locus of responsibility just present a new set of technical challenges, a new set of problems to be solved using the same methods that have proven effective in the past? Is future progress strictly a matter of figuring out how to effect changes in the host in the same way that we can now clean up the environment and subdue bacterial agents?

Heart disease, cancer, and strokes are now the three leading causes of death in the United States. Smoking, blood pressure, cholesterol levels, obesity, lack of exercise, alcohol misuse, and poor diet are the most significant risk factors for these diseases. Further reductions in heart disease will require reducing smoking, obesity, and inactivity. How are we going to do this? There is mixed evidence that diet pills may be effective in reducing obesity. Is the purpose of health promotion research to find even more effective behavior modification techniques, which can then be disseminated to skillfully trained health promotion specialists in the field?

The major risk factors for injuries, cirrhosis, suicide, and homicide are the misuse of alcohol and firearms. How are we supposed to think about intervening to control such risk factors? Pneumonia is caused by pneumococcal bacteria that can be treated with antibiotics. Is the point of health promotion to devise equally powerful techniques for controlling the causes of alcohol misuse? Is it the same sort of technical, scientific problem? Granted it may be more complicated and comparably effective behavioral interventions have not yet been discovered, but is this how we should be thinking about the means and ends of the field?

Acquired immunodeficiency syndrome is transmitted through unsafe sexual and drug injection practices. Researchers are actively seeking to find out how to arrest or mitigate the effects of the virus. Other researchers are just as strenuously trying to find out how to stop or limit unsafe sexual and drug injection practices. Is there anything different in their respective approaches? Isn't the primary objective of social scientists to find the behavioral equivalents of protease inhibitors?

Currently in the field of health promotion, there is no difference in the types of research funded by the federal government and most private foundations. The objectives and methods of behavioral research are identical to the objectives and methods of biological research. All research protocols supported by the NIH are subjected to the same review processes and the same standards that have been established in order to yield what is now considered valid, scientifically warranted knowledge. The fact that the genesis of modern maladies lies in the social milieu has produced no change in the basic research strategies that guide the field.

The shortcomings of the current approach arise because there is a qualitatively distinct dimension to the human condition not found in the natural world. The current direction in the field fails to recognize or appreciate the difference between biological processes and social practices. Social pathologies are "treated" just like physiological disease processes, in both senses of the word. The issues are defined in the same manner, as technical scientific problems to be solved. And scientists are trying to come up with "treatments" for social pathologies in the same way that they have developed cures for infectious diseases.

But modern maladies are primarily social in origin. They are largely due to disturbances in the sociocultural environment and the choices people make about how they want to live their lives. That these choices now lead to premature death is extremely interesting and important. One might even say there is something sick or pathological about the levels of drug abuse, homicide, suicide, child abuse, teen pregnancy, infant mortality, obesity, alcoholism, smoking, and drunk-driving deaths now found in our society. But their social origins create new and distinct challenges for the field of health promotion.

So, how should we think about solving the health and social problems in communities like Holyoke? Does a science of health promotion offer the best prospects for their remediation? Most students enter graduate school expecting that the health promotion program will impart the skills and competencies needed to prevent these problems effectively. What skills do public health promotion professionals working at the Holyoke Health Center, the Care Center, or Nueva Esperanza need to reduce AIDS, substance abuse, teen pregnancy, or infant mortality? Should health promotion professionals expect to gain skills to prevent someone from deciding to try drugs that are comparable to the skills that clinicians learn about how to administer medications to prevent heart attacks? Should they learn how to measure hypothesized risk factors in baseline surveys to identify the most strategic intervention points for behavior modification? Does it matter if it is their neighbor's behavior that they are targeting? How should they think about poverty or racism—as risk factors for which they are gaining the technical skills to address, or as political problems outside the sphere of their professionals concerns? How should they respond to the taxpayers' reluctance to fund programs at the health department because they are perceived as primarily serving poor people and people of color and not the majority population? What types of skills are training programs imparting to help students learn how to address the City Council's opposition to needle exchange programs, or the School Committee's opposition to sex education? Are these issues outside the scope of their professional responsibilities? Or is changing their behavior any different from changing a potential drug abuser's behavior? As a teacher, I think about these issues constantly. I do not think that science can solve the health problems people have in Holyoke. I think I do my students a disservice to go on as if scientific breakthroughs that will give them the power to change people's behaviors are near at hand. So what other resources do we have to call upon for addressing Holyoke's ills? I want to suggest that figuring out why Holyoke and the nation at large have such high levels of modern maladies and what people want to do about them are fundamentally ethical and political matters. After exploring the shortcomings of the scientific approach in greater detail, we examine the possibilities for another type of health promotion practice in Holyoke in the second half of this book.

3

THE LIMITS OF SCIENCE

> *Nam et ipsa scientia potestas est.*
> Knowledge is power.
> —Francis Bacon, *Meditationes Sacrae*, 1597

My students are invariably struck by the disparity between the results of health promotion research and research in other health science disciplines in terms of explanatory power. Not only do the standard health promotion theories appear incapable of predicting health-related behaviors, but they rarely rise above the commonplaces of human experience: people who have more confidence in their ability are more likely to take action than people who are less confident (self-efficacy); people who think they are going to get a disease are more likely to take action than people who think they are not going to get a disease (perceived susceptibility). Many students assume that the reason the results are not better is that researchers in health promotion are not as capable as other scientists. In fact, interventions are perceived to be so ineffective that health education has become something of the laughingstock of the health sciences. I set off on this intellectual journey wondering why this state of affairs had come to pass.

One starting point for thinking about the limits of the scientific method in explaining health behavior is to acknowledge this striking, surprising lack of success. Yet advocates maintain that the current approach is on course. Glanz, Lewis, and Rimer, for example, write, "the field is still relatively young,"[1] implying that, given more time and additional grant support, researchers will eventually come up with explanations and interventions on par with those found in the medical sciences. This chapter explains why a science of health promotion is neither imminent nor estimable.

The fact that experimental research designs work well in explaining biological processes in the human body poses particular challenges for researchers in health promotion. Health lies on the border between the natural and social worlds. The natural processes that determine physical health can now be explained with unprecedented power and precision through the use of the scientific method; the social practices that underlie individual and community well-being are not amenable to the same methods of analysis.[2] That natural processes and social practices intersect in the generation of human well-being complicates its study. To achieve a better understanding of how we might promote individual and community well-being will require a better balance between scientific, hypothesis-testing methods and more humanistic forms of research.[3] But because medical science has produced such effective interventions to control disease processes, there is strong resistance to the idea that different goals, methods, and assumptions might be necessary to come to terms with socially generated health problems.[4] The resistance is quite understandable, but ultimately also quite deleterious.

I come at the question of the limits of the scientific method from two tacks: first, by outlining historical shifts in what is considered valid knowledge and the evolution of the idea that knowledge should be equated with determining the causes of events; second, by describing several unique features of the human condition, and hence, what has been lost in this historical transition. In the final section, I show how the commitment to causal explanations contributes to the sense of modern moral malaise.

HISTORICAL SHIFTS IN EPISTEMOLOGY

Taylor claims that there has been a shift in the scope and warrants of reasoning in the modern era: "reason is no longer defined substantively, in terms of a vision of the cosmic order, but formally, in terms of the procedures thought ought to follow."[5] In outlining this historical shift in epistemology, I will be tracing one line in the ascent of instrumental reason. After describing this transformation, we will be able to see how this shift has led to a change in the way researchers think about human behavior. The standard procedures of the scientific method frame the kinds of questions that are asked about human behavior, casting them in terms of causes, rather than their meaning or morality. Because of the kinds of answers these types of questions yield, this transformation has led to the adoption of an instrumental stance—how to effect change—toward others and the world.

When Taylor argues that "modern reason tends to be understood no longer substantively but procedurally,"[6] I take him to be saying that the way we think about the world and what we mean when we claim we know some truth about it has changed. A chronicle of this transformation goes something like this. In the premodern world, the human capacity to reason meant to try to fathom God's will and to reflect on the best life for human beings and on how social institutions would need to be organized in order for people to live more closely attuned to this ideal. Scholars would flesh out ideas about prospective alternatives and rely on the coherence and cogency of their account to inspire people to act accordingly. One thinks of Plato's *Republic* as the classic example.

In the modern era, dating from the time of the Enlightenment, a well-known and readily traceable line of thinkers discovered (invented?) a set of procedures that, when followed, enabled them to make astonishingly accurate predictions. Over time, these procedures gradually became the basis for claiming one truly knew something about the world, that a particular claim was not just an opinion, an unwarranted assertion, or superstitious belief but that it was, in fact, *true*. So, with the rise of this way of thinking about things, when someone would make a statement about the world, the modern mind sought to recast the claim in ways whereby it could be tested and verified using these procedures. If it could be so recast, this framework then provided the criteria for determining its truth or error. Moreover, these criteria were formulated such that the capacity to effect change was inherent in their employment. They yielded power over the world. Let me be more concrete.

Writing at the beginning of the seventeenth century, Sir Francis Bacon's self-proclaimed mission was to purge the intellect of what he called "idols of the mind," mankind's presumptuous illusions and tendencies to error.[7] He wanted to eliminate erroneous thinking, expressly in order to gain mastery over nature. In his *Novum Organon* (1620), he set out to displace Aristotle's *Organon*, the premodern bible on science, through laying out a new system of inductive logic, the systematic collection of empirical and experimental data, and examples of the efficacy of this new approach. Bacon himself was not much of a scientist, but his writings were tremendously influential over the thought of Robert Boyle, Isaac Newton, and others. It would be remiss not to mention René Descartes and the considerable influence of his *Discourse on the Method of Rightly Conducting One's Reason and Seeking the Truth in the Sciences* (1637) too.

Born in 1627, Boyle is best known for his discovery of the ideal gas law, $PV = nRT$. So here is an assertion: the pressure of a gas in a closed container varies directly with its temperature. This statement can be recast as a hypothesis: If the temperature goes up, then the pressure will go up. The hypothesis can then be tested by increasing the temperature and observing what happens. Following these procedures, Boyle discovered he could unerringly predict what would happen to the pressure when he increased the temperature. And the very methods that he used to verify his claim gave him the ability to make the pressure do whatever he wanted.

This was heady stuff. When Bacon wrote in 1597, "Knowledge is power," he was not saying that scholarship bestowed prestige or gained one entree into the royal courts. He meant it in a more literal sense. He was saying that it is the power to effect change that *constitutes* knowledge. They are one and the same. (*Nam et ipsa scientia potestas est.*) People could claim they knew something for sure if they could demonstrate they knew how to effect change precisely as predicted. Over time, people came to believe that the criteria of prediction and control were the only way to know whether a statement was true or not. These procedures are what we now call the scientific method.

It is easy to see why people were won over to this new way of thinking. Consider the difference between Hippocrates's meditation on *Airs, Waters, and Places* and Koch's Postulates. Hippocrates's work is a prime example of how people went about explaining the world in the premodern era: hot and cold winds, the weight of water, how a town lies to the rising and setting sun. People went right on getting sick and dying and there did not seem to be much that anyone could do about it. Then, along come Robert Koch and Louis Pasteur who say they know what is making people sick and how to stop it. And they did.

Isaiah Berlin has suggested that the Enlightenment was inspired by a constellation of three supreme confidences: that all questions have one and only one true answer; that there is one and only one path to the discovery of these truths; and that, when found, these truths will all be compatible with one another.[8] Downstream, the dream of the Enlightenment has not lost its appeal. We are still buoyed by the promise of one path leading to the discovery of one truth. Taylor's claim is that this solitary path to knowledge is now blazed with procedural criteria. The credibility we give claims is directly proportional to the degree to which they have satisfied the criteria identified by Bacon and his descendants. The closer a particular claim fulfills these procedural guarantees, the more reasonable it seems; and conversely, the less one can show that some claim has been tested and verified, the less reasonable it seems.

But Taylor reminds us that this is not the only way of making sense of the world:

> Technological payoff, or the greater ability to predict and manipulate things, is certainly a good criterion of scientific success on the post-Galilean paradigm of understanding. If understanding is knowing your way about, then modern technological success is a sure sign of progress in knowledge. But how is this meant to convince a pre-Galilean? For in fact he is operating with a different paradigm of understanding, to which manipulative capacity is irrelevant, which instead proves itself through a different ability, that of discovering our proper place in the cosmos and finding attunement with it. . . . Each theory carries with it its own built-in criteria of success—moral vision and attunement in one case, manipulative power in the other—and is therefore invulnerable to the other's attack. In the end, we all seem to have gone for manipulative power, but this has to be for some extra-epistemic consideration, not because this mode of science has been shown to be superior as *knowledge*.[9]

Despite irreconcilable differences in their respective criteria for claiming knowledge, as the full power and benefits of the scientific method came to be more widely appreciated, researchers increasingly sought to reframe questions in terms of causality, questions for which hypotheses could be tested, in order to establish conclusive answers. On the other side of this same coin, the historian Joyce Appleby and her colleagues note that the principal legacy of the rise of the scientific worldview is an enduring belief in a firm dichotomy between objective knowledge and subjective opinion.[10] Claims not subjected to tests of verification have come to be regarded as unscientific, and from there, the logic and perceived superiority of this system of thought persistently press toward regarding them as baseless, unwarranted interjections.

A perceived dichotomy between objective scientific knowledge and subjective opinion is evident in the state of health promotion research today. To obtain grant funding and to publish in professional journals, one has to satisfy certain well-known procedural criteria: null hypotheses, operational definitions, tests of scale reliability and validity, random assignment, interrater reliability, statistical tests of significance appropriate to the level of measurement (nominal, ordinal, interval), calculations of statistical power, p-values, and the like. The prospects for securing grant support and the credibility of findings are directly related to the degree to which these criteria are met. The prestige of journals is proportional to the degree to which these standards are upheld; reviewers for the most prestigious journals consign anything less to the category of commentary, suitable only as editorial or opinion pieces.[11] While a few people, particularly practitioners, have voiced dissatisfaction with the results of research produced through rigorous adherence to these procedural standards (the "rigor-versus-relevance" debate), there is not a great deal of agreement about what a viable alternative might look like. Qualitative research has gained modest acceptance in recent years, but this is largely because it is readily subsumed under exploratory "hypothesis-generating" (Stage I) research and not because it represents a different kind of knowledge or might serve different purposes besides prediction and control.[12] With this background, we are now in a better position to survey the epistemological shortcomings and ethical pitfalls of the quest for a science of health promotion.

EPISTEMOLOGICAL SHORTCOMINGS

Against the current of this modern procedural/scientific stream of thought, another long line of philosophers has observed, defined, and defended the idea that there are categorically distinct features of the human condition that make knowledge about social reality irreducible to the kind of knowledge obtained in the natural sciences. In an exposition that in many respects has never been surpassed, Aristotle introduced the idea in the *Nichomachean Ethics*. There, Aristotle describes three types of knowledge, corresponding to three different types of experience.[13]

The first type of experience Aristotle observed is the experience of events that are constant, universal, and eternal; these experiences occur in the encounter with the natural world. Aristotle termed this sphere of experience *theoria* and knowledge about it *episteme*. Aristotle's second category refers to the experience of making things—know-how or craftsmanship. He termed this experience *poesis* and the type of knowledge appropriate to it, *techne*. The third type of experience comes from the encounter with flux: the transient, irregular, context-bound, and contingent relationships characteristic of the sociohistorical domain. He called this kind of experience *praxis* and the corresponding knowledge *phronesis*, or practical reason.

Based on Aristotle's original distinctions, there are (at least) three major lines of philosophical thought that have evolved over time describing the unique qualities of human action that defy causal analysis, in effect arriving at the same conclusion coming from different angles. (This literature is vast. I can only introduce the main lines of argument in these brief summaries and hope that they will be inviting enough to encourage readers to delve into the issues in greater depth on their own.) I will call these three lines of argument: (*1*) the openness of the social world; (*2*) human agency (free will); and, (*3*) the problem of meaning, or the linguistic foundations of social reality.

Openness of the Social World

Aristotle identified three features of social interactions that make scientific knowledge (*episteme*) inadequate and inappropriate for analyzing social situations: mutability, indeterminacy, and particularity. The classics scholar Martha Nussbaum elaborates on Aristotle's ideas, noting that in contrast to the constant cause-and-effect relationships typically found between objects in the natural world, Aristotle observed that human relationships are historical, contextual, and contingent. Action in the social domain must be responsive to the novel features of each situation, to contexts in which a limitless variety of features fluctuate in salience, and to the ethical relevance of the particular persons in the specific situation at hand.[14]

While the force of gravity is uniform throughout the known universe (except, possibly, in black holes), Aristotle noted that relationships in the sociohistorical domain do not display the same invariability. On the contrary, how people respond to events depends on when and where they occur, who is present, and what the individuals hope to accomplish. Social events transpire in the context of nonrecurring, singular configurations of actors and elements. Also, individuals can and do revise their perceptions of the (most) relevant features of any given situation, leading to variable responses. More broadly, the values we consider important change over time as do our interpretations of the meaning of those values. By way of contrast, to imagine the recurrence of the same circumstances with the same persons in the very same state of mind is to imagine a world that does not exist.[15]

Social situations are inherently indeterminate. The potential features of a situation that may be picked out and may have bearing on a decision are in principle inexhaustible. Not only is there change over time (which introduces the element of surprise), but the relevance of different ingredients depends on the context of events. Moreover, different actors attending the same situation may consider different elements more or less pertinent and act on their subjective perceptions of what is pertinent to them at that time, making any attempt at an objective cataloguing of factors impossible. Finally, social relationships are defined in terms of their particularity. Aristotle is referring here specifically to the ethical relevance of the particular people present; each person is a unique individual with whom we have a unique relationship, unique feelings, and a unique history of mutual acquaintance.

Aristotle thought scientific knowledge was inadequate for analyzing social situations because life is such that we are confronted with the need to make decisions regarding the best course of action at *this* time in *this* specific spot, in all its mutable, indeterminate, and particular complexity. Viewed from this vantage point, human behavior is unpredictable to the extent that decisions are based on recognition of the unique features of each particular situation.[16]

Human Agency

A second line of argument involves the human capacity for agency, or free will. The question of free will has not finally been resolved one way or the other in philosophical circles, but the main contours of the argument in favor of the possibility run along these lines.[17]

For Aristotle, the principal evidence that human reactions are not determined by prior events is the primal observation that human choices, in his words, "could be other than they are." He continues, "For where it is in our power to act, it is also in our power not to act, and where we can say 'no,' we can also say 'yes.' "[18] Plainly, if there is any fact of experience that we are all familiar with, it is the simple fact that our own choices seem to make a difference in our actual behavior. There are all sorts of experiences where it seems just a fact of our experience that though we did one thing, we know perfectly well that we could have done something else.[19] Kant likewise drew a sharp line between the physical sciences and moral reasoning. In Kant's terms, the natural world is governed by necessity, whereas the social world is the realm of will, intentionality, and freedom.[20]

More recently, to introduce another distinction frequently cited in the literature, von Wright described the difference between scientific explanation and humanistic understanding.[21] Von Wright argued that human behavior can never be adequately explained in causal terms, but must also be understood teleologically, i.e., in terms of purposive, value-laden, goal-directed will, volition, and intentions. A complete account of human behavior can never be achieved by searching for antecedent causes if people have the capacity to choose among future courses of action. Chemicals mixed in a test tube do not decide what they want to do. People do, they make choices. Because of this ability, people are not prisoners of the past. Unlike events in nature, human action is not inexorably driven by antecedent causes.

People look for reasons for choosing one course of action over another. Over and above (and often in spite of) the force of antecedent causes, human beings have the unique capacity to pursue prospective goals divined through an imaginative, critical consciousness and tempered by a moral conscience. To make a conscious decision is an act of will. People transcend their past personal experiences through resolving to be better persons. Human projects look forward, hoping to realize—to bring into being—ideals of a better world. The assumption that there are causes that force people to act in predictable ways denies the creative quality of the human mind. People live in the world as active subjects, not merely as passive objects.[22] To search exclusively for the presumed antecedent causes thus misses at least half the picture, looking only at the past, not at the future. For researchers, whenever one sees regular, consistent patterns of behavior, it is important to remember the different assumptions and different implications entailed between thinking that social norms "cause" certain behaviors and recognizing that people may choose to uphold social norms for reasons having to do with a deliberate identification with a valued, shared way of social life.

Based on the standard set by the verification principle, positivist research methodologies are limited to the search for causes. Health researchers who believe randomized control trials provide the highest standard of scientific proof must then proceed on the assumption that health-related behaviors can be adequately explained by identifying and verifying their presumed antecedent causes. The possibility that human beings might possess the capacity for agency is considered moot.[23] Clearly, human behavior is influenced by the past; our decisions are undoubtedly affected in subtle and often unconscious ways by past experience. The strong, consistent association between health status and income suggests that there are indeed socioeconomic constraints on the degree to which people can exercise free choice. But causal explanations can be considered sufficient for understanding human behavior only if one rejects the possibility of free will, an assumption worth questioning.

The Problem of Meaning

Finally, in the most influential line of thought, the shortcomings of the positivist system were decisively brought to light by the "linguistic turn" in philosophy.[24] According to this philosophical school, the most important difference between the human condition and the natural world arises through the human ability to use language. As a result of this unique human ability, there is a categorical onto-logical difference between social practices and natural processes. The essence of social practices is not embedded in the structure of matter, but lies in the language that human beings use to generate and interpret their meaning. Social practices do not have an objective existence independent of the language by which we choose to describe them. In Taylor's terms, while natural processes are independent of the language used to describe them, social practices are *constituted* by the very language that is used to describe them.[25]

To illustrate, in the natural world, the orbiting of the moon is caused by the force of gravity. The moon will continue to orbit whether or not we care to de-scribe what it is doing. Moreover, however we choose to describe the orbiting of the moon, it has no effect on the moon's behavior. Whether we say it is due to "gravity" or due to "phlogiston," the moon goes on orbiting just the same. But social practices are not independent of their description.[26]

Taylor offers the example of "voting" to explain the difference. Voting is a social practice; it is a collective act by which decisions are made. In New England town meetings, the practice is carried out through raising hands. But, unlike the orbit-ing of the moon, the act of voting cannot take place unless we define what we mean by this peculiar social practice. The critical insight of the linguistic turn is that social practices, such as voting, are not independent of the language we use to describe them. This revelation has profound implications for the study of human behavior.

When we set out to conduct research on human behavior, we find that the act of hand raising does not have objective, language-independent determinants. That is, the "cause" of people raising their hands depends on the meaning people give to the act. To highlight this dependence, we need only think of other contexts: school children raise their hands to get called upon by their teacher, football players raise their hands to signal a fair catch, other people raise their hands to say hello. What is the "cause" of hand-raising behavior? It depends on what they are doing. But what they are doing can only be known through the words we use to describe and give meaning to the act. Human behavior is motivated by reasons that are inexorably tied to the language we use to make sense of our existence.[27]

In this perspective, human behavior can be, and often is, motivated by under-standings of the kind of life one wants to live, the kind of person one wants to be, the kind of society one wants to live in, and the concomitant effort of will exerted to realize those values, to lead the kind of life one thinks best under given circum-stances.[28] Here, the motivation itself is an act of interpretive understanding be-cause the ideas themselves are a product of the creative human imagination. They are not "out there" inscribed in the structure of the universe. Our understanding of justice is constituted by the language we use to define and debate about it; it is not something that exists independently, outside of the words we use to make sense of it. Values are neither subjective nor objective but interpersonal. We cannot just make them up as we go along, but neither are they etched indelibly into the natural order. They exist in a historical sociocultural medium, transmitted from one generation to the next, in which interpretations change and evolve over time. People are born into a world in which understandings about values always already exist, but these understandings are also always subject to revision and further clarification. Attempts to impose operational definitions on values as if they were objective, language-neutral forces of nature that could be measured like gravity are thus deceptive, misleading, and inappropriate.

To take an example closer to home, "well-being" is understood by some people to be a state that is achieved through proper diet and exercise. For others, "well-being" is understood to be a state that is achieved through acting on one's social conscience: being courageous, living modestly, pursuing justice, and aspiring to wisdom. Here is the critical point. Unlike the moon, people's behavior is motivated by their take on the concept. What sorts of prescriptions health promoters deliver depend on what they understand well-being to be. What people will do depends on their understanding of what they hope to accomplish. Unlike descriptions of natural processes, there is no neutral, objective, independent description that can reconcile these different interpretations and determine what well-being "really" is. How we choose to describe human behavior and human motivation makes a difference. Meanings are created, challenged, and fought over during the course of history and human events. This ontological difference between natural processes and social practices creates intractable problems for a methodology based on the assumption that it is possible to give objective, value-free descriptions.[29]

There is one more vitally important point that follows from the unique capacity of human beings to use language. It is the ability to use language that gives people the capacity for ethical conduct, the capacity for acting with autonomy and responsibility. Unlike other creatures, human beings can evaluate options and choose different courses of action based on their understanding of the kind of life human beings ought to live. We can choose, in a way animals and inanimate objects cannot. Human beings have the singular ability to be responsible for what they think is good for them. "What is distinctively human," Taylor points out, "is the power to evaluate our desires, to regard some as desirable and others are [sic] undesirable."[30]

Human beings alone have the ability to discriminate and make judgments about the quality of their appetites. According to Taylor,

> Human beings are not alone in having desires and motives, or in making choices. They share these things with members of certain species, some of which even appear to engage in deliberation and to make decisions based on prior thought. It seems to be peculiarly characteristic of humans, however, that they are able to form . . . second-order desires. . . . Our [first-order] desires are classified in such categories as higher and lower, virtuous and vicious, more or less fulfilling, more or less re-

fined, profound and superficial, noble and base. They are judged as belonging to qualitatively different modes of life: fragmented or integrated, alienated or free, saintly or merely human, courageous or pusillanimous, and so on. . . . In the first case, which we may call weak evaluation, we are concerned with outcomes; in the second, strong evaluation, with the quality of our motivation. . . . Strong evaluation is concerned with the qualitative *worth* of different desires.[31]

Like animals, human beings experience first-order felt desires (to eat, to drink, to have sex, etc.), but then the human race has the distinctive ability to evaluate the quality of these appetites, judging them worthy of pursuing or not, thus forming second-order desires about human conduct. Our capacity for moral responsibility is intimately, inextricably bound up with this ability to make second-order strong evaluations of felt desires.

Stuart Hampshire provides one final example illustrating the implications of the linguistic turn in philosophy. Phenomenologically, whether or not human beings "really" have the capacity for agency, the fact that people think that they have the capacity for making choices and that these "choices could be other than they are" makes the quest for objective accounts illusory. As we reflect on what we did, we often change our interpretation of events based on what we think we should have done, and so change the nature of the experience. In Hampshire's revealing example,

A person may make moral judgments of many different kinds about the past: that he ought to have chosen differently at various junctures; or that he ought to have foreseen some of the worst outcomes. . . . He explains himself to himself by his history, but by the history as accompanied by unrealized possibilities on both sides of the track of actual events. His individual nature, and the quality of his life, do not depend only on the bare log-book of events and actions. His character and the quality of his experience emerge in the possibilities that were real possibilities for him, which he considered and rejected for some reason or other.[32]

In this light, a strictly objective specification of actual empirical antecedent events is plainly lacking in terms of understanding the nature of human experience. The meaning of events emerges in large part in reflections about what we think we should or might have done too. The language of moral reflection shapes our experience of what "actually" happened.

In sum, from an epistemological standpoint, what has been lost in the transition to the positivist system of verification is everything that makes us uniquely human. The commitment of health promotion researchers to explaining human behavior in terms of cause-and-effect relationships has created a void in our understanding of human behavior. What is missing from these explanations is the human ability to discern different meanings in the past, to imagine different futures, to choose the values by which we think we ought to live, and to create a life on the basis of the will to become the kind of people we deem worthy. What is missing is any appreciation of the bases of human autonomy, responsibility, dignity, and respect. As the philosopher Charles Larmore concludes: "We need to recognize how the world is not exhausted by what the sciences can tell us of it. Reality also contains a normative dimension, constituted by reasons for belief and action."[33]

To bring the two preceding sections together, in light of the significant accomplishments of modern science, NIH-funded health researchers, in general, use the same analytic methods and research designs (i.e., RCTs) to investigate human behavior that they use to examine physiological reactions. But, as a consequence, the field of health promotion finds itself struggling to make do with findings such as the following.

After 30 years of intensive research into the causes of youthful substance abuse, a prominent team of highly regarded researchers summarizes progress to date: "The major risk factors for drug abuse in adolescence may be classified into three categories: behavioral, social, and demographic. Consistently the strongest predictor of drug use has been past use. The strongest social predictors have been use by adolescents' parents and friends, and the most consistent demographic predictors have been age and gender."[34] In other words, after millions of dollars of research, we now know that older males who have already tried drugs themselves and whose parents and friends use drugs are, in general, more likely to use drugs than teens who have never tried drugs, who are younger, female, and whose parents and friends do not use drugs. When I read statements like these, I worry about the state of my profession. As long as certain procedural criteria have been met, no one seems bothered by the fact that, substantively, the results are trivial. While one example does not make the case, it is illustrative of the problems besetting efforts to establish the scientific foundations of health promotion.[35] Criticisms of the quality of results found in these types of social scientific studies transcend ideological boundaries too. Scholars and pundits from across the political spectrum—liberal,[36] radical,[37] and conservative[38]—have expressed similar dismay.

The shortcomings of such studies arise because researchers are asking the wrong questions. The political philosopher William Sullivan observes that the rise of the scientific worldview has displaced the focus of research—from questions about the ends, meaning, or values that guide human behavior to a search for its presumed antecedent causes.[39] Ian Angus characterizes the conversion in this way: "The transformation from the classical question 'why' things are as they are to the modern 'how.'"[40] Researchers do not ask why people pursue activities that may harm their health in an attempt to reveal what these activities may mean to them or why they might think the choices they have made are more or less fulfilling for them in light of their circumstances. They ask instead how it happens—what causes these unhealthy behaviors—and how can they be prevented. The principal shortcoming of the scientific research agenda for health promotion is the failure to pursue questions about the meaning or morality of behavior, questions that might help us gain greater clarity about different values, their relative merit, and insight into how their competing claims might be resolved in specific situations.

Scientific research does not pursue questions about meaning, morality, or values because they cannot be empirically verified. There is no scientific basis—no hypotheses to be tested—for determining the validity of these kinds of value claims: whether it is worth sacrificing one's (physical) health for a social cause; or whether high levels of poverty and inequality are morally acceptable (whether or not they are associated with poor health status); or whether a life of caring for others is more worthwhile than a life given over to the pursuit of self-interests (e.g., Is exercising for 3 hours per week more worthwhile than volunteering at a community shelter for 3 hours per week?); or whether teenagers can have sexual relations in ways consistent with our understanding of what it means to be a good human being, to lead a decent life, to grow to be the kind of person we admire and want them to be; or whether individuals should be free to decide for themselves if they want to try marijuana, or whether all of the state's resources should be marshaled to devise the most powerful and effective techniques possible to eliminate the desire to try it. The scientific method is incapable of answering questions about any such substantive value claims.

As a result, the field is caught up in this strange enterprise where researchers seeking to develop a science of health promotion go on as if these issues were immaterial since they cannot be subjected to scientific analysis. The skew is apparent in perusing any NIH research grant announcement or health promotion journal. Articles addressing normative issues, such as the priority of different human values, the meaning and significance of different visions of the good life for human beings, or qualitative distinctions of worth among different ideals about how we should live are absent, invisible. Because the scientific method is incapable of addressing such questions, the predominant orientation of the field is to pursue other lines of inquiry, forging ahead as if research into the meaning and morality of behavior was not necessary for understanding why people make the choices they do.

To put this another way, the scientific method is unsurpassable at determining the direction and magnitude of relationships if and when they are causal in nature, "A causes B." These methods do not work well when the nature of the relationship is not exhausted by causal characterizations. To recall an example from the previous chapter, teenagers may indeed experience low self-esteem, but they still have choices about how they want to act in light of their experience and self-understanding. The scientific method meets its limit here. It has nothing to offer in response to their questions about the kind of life they may want to lead, the kind of person they want to be, or why one way of living might be more esteemed than another. It can only determine whether or not, if one pumps up their level of self-esteem, then lower levels of drug use may (or may not) be more likely.

Critics suggest it is the failure to attend to the crucial ontological differences in the human condition that explains why the scientific method has consistently been shown to account for such small amounts of the variability in human behavior. Because social practices are not fixed, immutable, or structured into the fabric of the universe, but instead must be intentionally willed, based, at least in part, on one's interpretation of human values and ethical principles, the quest for discovering causal relationships will never suffice for understanding human behavior. In the end, the major epistemological shortcoming of the positivist scientific method is that it does not work, on its own terms. Despite ample opportunity, it has not given researchers the power to predict human behavior.

Finally, a better appreciation of the epistemological shortcomings of the positivist paradigm might bring to a close a question that has perennially vexed the field. The alleged gap between theory and practice arises not because proven theories are too abstruse for practitioners to comprehend, but because they are too limited, the results too banal.[41] Because of its failure to take into account that which makes us uniquely human, the results typically reproduce simple truisms, repackaged in academic jargon. Because of its shortcomings, the most powerful explanations of health behavior that the conventional approach has been able to produce are findings like "people who think that disease X is more severe are more likely to take action than people who think it is less severe." These kinds of outcomes result from the commitment to a system of thought that assumes behavior can be adequately explained as the product of antecedent causes.

ETHICAL PITFALLS

Because of its epistemological shortcomings, the ethical pitfalls of the scientific framework for health promotion are not what one might expect at first glance. The most commonly voiced ethical concern about applied social scientific research revolves around the potential for coercion and manipulation of behavior.[42] But no matter how much more time, money, and effort are invested, the field of health promotion will never develop this power, I think, for reasons discussed above. Human creativity routinely defies prediction and control. Instead, the ethical pitfalls result from how an instrumental mindset leads us to think about human progress in general and the means and ends of health promotion in particular. The scientific orientation of the field frames the way we think about our relationships to others. It fosters the idea that the purpose of health promotion is to seek and to wield the power necessary to effect changes in other people's behaviors. It defines our relationship to one another in terms of trying to figure out how to get others to do what we want them to do, rather than in terms of trying to reach common understandings about the good life for human beings.

As we saw in the first chapter, Taylor and other scholars are deeply concerned about the rise of instrumental reason, the modern preoccupation with devising ever more effective techniques to the neglect and abandonment of reflection on ends. This bias is evident in the perceived superiority of procedural, cause-and-effect scientific thinking over other modes of human inquiry. Because of the way its internal standards are set up, the scientific method gives answers to questions about the means to an end: the causes that produce an effect. The skew is inherent in the formulation of hypotheses (the "if–then" criterion), the search for causes, and the standards of prediction and control. By the same token, the scientific method cannot answer questions about the intrinsic worthiness of different values or purposes. Substantive questions about the value of different pursuits are beyond the capability of hypothesis-testing methods. Based on what it can and cannot do, the scientific method is thus inherently instrumental. How then does the commitment to developing a science of health promotion contribute to the malaise and decline in values perceived by pundits surveying the state of health and social conditions in modern America?

To reiterate, Taylor argues that individualism and instrumental reason are the two primary sources of modern malaise, the perplexing sense of loss, decline, and disintegration felt in contemporary culture. Taylor and others see many distinct problems emerging from the rise of an instrumental worldview. I want to sketch out a short list of these consequences here. Again, I do not want to suggest that the quest for a science of health promotion is responsible for all that troubles us these days; the field suffers from these larger cultural and intellectual currents as much as it perpetuates them. But it is important for those of us in the field to see more clearly the ways in which the direction we are now headed contributes to these larger problems. To the extent that the pursuit of a science of health promotion reinforces—or fails to challenge—the dominant instrumental ethos, the field adds its weight to the following problems: (*1*) the foundations of values are being undermined; (*2*) clarity about goals is being subordinated to the pursuit of more effective means; (*3*) the intrinsic value of various social practices is being eroded; (*4*) the relationship between means and ends misconstrued; and (*5*) respect for the dignity and autonomy of individuals threatened as the intent to effect change in others' behavior is promulgated. The current direction of the field of health promotion is not aimed at clarifying and strengthening values, but rather has fallen in line with the forces leading to their erosion.

Undermining the Foundations of Values

The primacy afforded procedural, instrumental thinking undermines the credibility of value claims. Relative to the accomplishments of modern science, discussions about meaning, morality, and the good for human beings seem to lack comparably objective criteria by which questions can be rationally resolved and firm conclusions drawn. Because positivists claim that certain procedural criteria must be met in order to ascertain truth, there are no "valid" methods of research for pursuing questions about the respective merits and worthiness of different values. The apparent lack of scientific procedures for testing and verifying their validity contributes to the perception or apprehension that value claims do not stand on solid grounds. And in an age when science has the franchise on determining whether propositions can be called true or not, value claims then appear to fall on the other side of the mental divide, with nowhere to go except into the residual category of subjective opinion. The essence of this predicament is that, if value statements do not count as objective, verifiable knowledge, then what are we to make of them? The bent of the modern mind presses toward regarding them as something less—less credible, less respectable, less warranted, less redeemable, less trustworthy. Absent verification, values seem to be little more than subjective preferences, impervious to the kinds of evidence that permit rational determinations. This state of affairs feeds the perception that there is no reasoned basis for ascertaining the common good and, hence, no recourse for resolving value disputes other than the clash of powers.

Researchers using the scientific method treat values empirically as subjective beliefs. The scientific method cannot answer questions about whether liberalism is good per se, but rather than considering alternative bases for rationally grounding such a claim (for example, through examining its historical origins or judging the quality of its ideas in comparison with other principles defining the good life for human beings[43]), researchers committed to testing hypotheses have little alternative but to treat such value claims as personal opinions. This individual holds these "liberal" beliefs, that one does not, and these are the behaviors that are associated with those beliefs. In one of the more egregious examples of the distortions caused by these methodological constraints, "liberalism" was operationally defined in a study of youthful drug abuse with the following four-item scale: "(*1*) support women's liberation—don't feel women need or want it, (*2*) see cops as law enforcers—see cops as 'pigs', (*3*) think police should carry guns—think cops shouldn't carry guns, and (*4*) approve of many protests—approve of few protests."[44] Despite its rich history in inspiring the American Revolution and framing the Declaration of Independence, the Constitution, and the Bill of Rights, liberalism is here defined as the belief that cops are pigs. (As the researchers, incidentally, found that "liberalism" correlated with higher levels of drug use, one could conclude that liberal beliefs should be reduced or eliminated.) In this type of research process, values are reduced to personal preferences arising from incorrigible individual gut feelings.

To the extent that institutional practices propagate the idea that the scientific method is the best or only means to validate claims about the world, discussions of values, purposes, and goals are relegated to a perceived unruly arena in which there are allegedly no objective criteria for deriving conclusions or adjudicating differences amidst the clash of personal preferences. When the NIH panel cited in the first chapter laments the intrusion of politics into AIDS treatment, they buttress this wall—there is science, and then there is nonscience. Against this view, Taylor argues that it is the distinctively human ability to evaluate our desires—to make rational, defensible, qualitative judgments of worth—that is undermined by the authority of the scientific method in the modern era. As we will see in Chapter 7, Sandel argues that this same penchant undermines our confidence in the possibility of achieving agreement about the common good, and thus, reinforces the assertion of procedural rights to protect self-interests.

Subordinating Questions about Goals to Questions about Means

Based on what the scientific method can and cannot do, questions focusing on determining the most effective means to an end take precedence over questions about the ends themselves. That is to say, more resources are allocated toward developing new treatment and prevention technologies than toward articulating, criticizing, broadening, or refining our understanding of human well-being. In concrete terms, researchers gain grant support to find out how to prevent substance abuse, not to study or investigate why drug use should or should not be allowed. Researchers are asked to develop more effective methods for preventing teen pregnancy, not to help adolescents articulate more clearly the value they see in having intimate relations (or, for that matter, to clarify the value in waiting). In Taylor's analysis, it is the rise of instrumental reason that is behind this characteristic tendency to give priority to questions about means over questions about ends.

What are the implications for the field of health promotion? In health promotion, an instrumental interest in maximizing efficiency permeates institutional thinking such that the logic of determining ends and means runs something like this. What is the most serious health problem? Death. What is the most common cause of death? Heart attacks. What is the most common cause of heart attacks? Smoking. Therefore, preventing cigarette smoking is the number one priority of the field. Although *Healthy People 2000* nominally identifies improving the quality of life as one goal, it is expected to be achieved through accomplishing much narrower risk reduction objectives. Currently, resources are overwhelmingly directed toward promoting biological fitness (lowering heart disease rates through prescriptions of nonsmoking, a strict diet, and regular exercise), rather than toward any broader goal of achieving individual or community well-being.

So, rather than wrestling with messy ethical and political questions about whether promoting social well-being might be more worthwhile than preventing heart disease, we find ourselves in a situation where the field has settled on certain objectives, as if by default, because they seem the most efficient. Reducing morbidity and mortality rates is expedient in defining operational objectives, which can be measured with the highest degree of accuracy and which enable researchers to calculate the effectiveness and efficiency of an intervention with the highest degree of precision possible, nowadays almost without question, quantitatively. Consequently, broader goals are left undone. But as a result, community members are left puzzled and frustrated as health promoters continue to stress smoking cessation, rather than issues the community members consider more important to their well-being, such as eliminating poverty, promoting equality, and improving the quality of our social institutions (schools, police departments, health care organizations, worksites, etc.).

Collapsing Intrinsic Values

Likewise, the intrinsic value of social practices is being discounted. It is becoming increasingly difficult to justify any activities except in instrumental terms, that is, except in terms of rationalizing them as a means to an end, and not as something valued in its own right. We saw earlier how one health education textbook consistently reverts to claims of effectiveness and cost-effectiveness. In health promotion, we aim to raise teenagers' self-esteem, not because that is good in its own right, but because it will result in lower drug use. More and more, health promotion activities as a whole are justified not on principle—not on the basis that people have a right to the information we provide and providing this information is valuable and important in and of itself in creating a society of informed consumers (whether or not it changes their behavior)—but because they will lower health care costs. Similarly, activists in the health field committed to the fight against poverty fall into the same instrumental mindset, claiming it is important not because the toleration of poverty is fundamentally wrong and unconscionable, but because it will reduce drug abuse, violence, and so on.

Misconstruing the Relationship between Means and Ends

When we think about issues in instrumental terms, means and ends are regarded as separate and independent issues. I touched on this point in the first chapter and will expand on those remarks here and again in Chapter 5.

One can get a picture of instrumental thinking about issues by considering the concept of "independent" variables as they are defined in the natural sciences. In Boyle's ideal gas law ($PV = nRT$), for example, the pressure can be increased by raising the temperature, increasing the number of moles of gas, or decreasing the volume. All will effectively change the pressure. Significantly, all can be defined and measured independently of one another. Definitions and measures of the temperature of a gas are separate from the definitions and measures of the volume, pressure, or number of moles of the gas.

When this way of thinking is applied to issues in the social domain, the processes that are used to select a particular end are considered separate and independent of the processes that are used to decide the most appropriate means of attaining that end. Who decides and why they decide weight control is important are considered separate and independent issues from the question of how weight control is to be achieved. Similarly, the instrumental bent presses toward considering different means of achieving health promotion goals as independent and interchangeable. To stop smoking, people can and do now undergo hypnosis, aversive conditioning, acupuncture, apply nicotine patches, substitute gum-chewing, or quit cold turkey. All are coming to be regarded as equally valid means of achieving the goal of smoking cessation, and again, the most important research question is to determine the most cost-efficient means to achieve the designated goal. To the extent that an instrumental, technical point of view is increasingly taking precedence over other considerations, health is increasingly coming to be seen as a product that can be produced, an outcome to be effected, in the same way that bridges can be built and men landed on the moon. It is a state that can be engineered through the operation of effective techniques.

In contrast, the proposal here is that well-being is a human value, not a discrete state that can be defined independently of the means used to get there. It is a certain way of living, a way of being in the world. As a human value, it is realized when people live with integrity, dignity, autonomy, and responsibility.

The difference in these perspectives goes back to a point raised earlier in this chapter. The problem with the objective, scientific view arises because it fails to take into account the fact that social practices are not independent of the language of description. In the natural world, matter and forces exist independently of the way we choose to describe them. But this is not the case with social practices. How we describe and characterize human purposes shapes human motivation. The ends are not independent of the means.

With the rise of instrumental reason, we have reduced individual well-being to physical fitness because it can be precisely measured and quantified (blood pressure, cholesterol counts, treadmill stress tests, etc.) and the levels of these indicators can be determined independently, irrespective of any information about the quality of a person's life. This framework enables scientists to transform health into a technical problem[45] of discovering the most effective means for lowering these indicators, again, in theory and in practice, independently from any consideration of the kind of life the individual is leading. So it seems we are well on the way toward developing drugs that will enable people to eat their cake but not have to wear it too. And on one level, restoring biophysiological functioning is strictly a matter of repairing or controlling physical breakdowns occurring in the natural order and the science of medicine works very well in this respect.

But on another level, the rise of instrumental reason has obscured the relationship between means and ends inherent in the social domain. In the social domain, gaining clarity about the value of some goal is an essential part of moving in that direction; means and ends cannot be divorced from one another. If we understand human dignity to be an essential part of human well-being, then the exercise of autonomy, responsibility, and self-control are inextricably intertwined in the process of realizing well-being. The ends of dignity and well-being are defined and constituted by the means of acting responsibly, choosing freely to exercise self-restraint in response to felt appetites because that is the kind of person one aspires to be, and caring for others because they share in and sustain our understanding of the dignity of human life. As weight loss centers increasingly succumb to prescribing diet pills and abandon a philosophy of responsible self-control, we lose sight of yet another source of the significance of living a human life, with its struggles, setbacks, and joys in overcoming adversity and temptation. When social problems are viewed as technical scientific problems best left to the experts, we abdicate our moral and political responsibility for improving the quality of our institutions. We will see more examples of the problems that arise when means and ends are viewed instrumentally in the next chapter.

Treating People as a Means to an End

The idea that the mission of health promotion is to effect change in other people's behavior constantly butts up against the fundamental ethical principle of respecting the dignity and autonomy of individuals. An ardent advocate, B. F. Skinner understood well the implications of developing a science of human behavior, titling his opus, *Beyond Freedom and Dignity*. Plans for meeting the nation's health objectives verge on designs that treat people as means to an end. Yet rather than reexamine current practices in the field and seriously consider alternative approaches, defenders of the scientific approach contend that there are sufficient ethical safeguards to prevent the field from manipulating people toward ends not of their own choosing.

An apt analogy here is the contraceptive technology of Norplant. Norplant changes the body's physiological functioning. Currently, the mainstream program of health promotion research seeks to prevent smoking and drug-taking with the same power, efficacy, and effectiveness that Norplant has to prevent pregnancy. Imagine if this line of research developed a truly effective technology for behavioral modification. To provide an example inspired by the results of an actual study,[46] an analogous prevention program might be to provide "conditioning in low-thought situations" in combination with catalytic medications, an intervention that effectively prevented people from forming the desire to take mind-altering drugs. What would it mean if these types of interventions were successfully developed? Bluntly, we might eliminate lifestyle diseases, but at a cost of desiccating that which makes human life meaningful. If successful, the quest would render meaningless the very concepts of human autonomy and responsibility. Clearly, this sort of effective intervention is not anywhere on the horizon, but nevertheless, this is still the direction the field is headed. It is what the current program of research is trying to accomplish.

I do not want to make too much of this point because I believe most health promotion professionals have a genuine regard for the welfare of the people they serve and see themselves as helping people to achieve goals that everyone considers worthwhile. As the ethical code for the field prescribes, effecting change is not problematic when participation is voluntary. But because public health takes a population-based approach (that is, we rarely intervene with individuals but instead target whole populations at a time), the degree to which everyone has agreed to the goals and fully understands the potential side effects of the procedures to which they will be subjected is dubious at best. When schools initiate drug prevention programs, have all students agreed that they want to stop using drugs and are only looking for assistance in achieving this goal? As health departments gear up their AIDS education programs, are community concerns (e.g., condom distribution in predominantly Catholic, Latino neighborhoods) ever subordinated to quarterly tallies of numbers served, as specified in their funding contract? When whole cities are selected for national intervention trials (22, in the case of COMMIT), did everyone know and approve of the treatment conditions? As the government moves forward with mass media campaigns to combat illegal drug use, who will insure that informed consent has been obtained before subjecting people to the most effective persuasive communication techniques money can buy? But, of course, it is hard to get too excited about these issues because the interventions themselves are so feeble.

Participation in these types of activities, however, does not work in the direction of fostering a stronger, clearer understanding of the fundamental dignity and autonomy of individuals. As the field becomes more engrossed with developing more effective techniques to eliminate illegal drug use or prevent teenage sexual activity, we forsake our responsibility to engage others in discussions about the good life for human beings, discussions aimed at expanding the sphere of consensus about the kinds of lives worth living and values worth upholding. Instead, the presumption is that we know what is in people's best interests better than they do themselves. Health educators are quick and proud to proclaim themselves "change agents." Yet it is hard to reconcile "selecting targets to effect behavior change" with the goal of promoting individual autonomy, if by autonomy one means, "To act for reasons of one's own and to take responsibility for those actions."[47] Because of the scientific ambitions of the field, we must make a conscious effort to remind ourselves of the necessary ethical precautions. Even on those occasions when target populations are invited to participate in program planning, we have to remind ourselves that we do it out of respect for community members as bearers of dignity and autonomy with the right to self-determination, and not because research has shown community participation to be more effective and more likely to produce greater change.[48]

In the end, my concern is that, as the field embraces the idea of a science of health promotion and drills professionals in this approach, the inherent instrumental biases will not be made explicit and other ways of thinking about the means and ends of health promotion will not be entertained. Without more serious consideration of other viable alternatives, the potential for treating people as a means to an end looms larger and more difficult to resist. Finally, even with voluntary consent, I fear the field has little appreciation of the deleterious assumptions underlying current social scientific theories, issues we will explore in the next chapter.

The German philosopher Friedrich Nietzsche was profoundly disturbed by "the nihilistic consequences of our natural sciences"[49] and he prophesied that modernity would increasingly be characterized by the will to power. If there is no perceived objective basis for making substantive value claims, if values are regarded as merely matters of subjective opinion and personal preferences, then it is in one's interest to have the power to make sure one's preferences prevail. Casting his eyes over the same terrain, the philosopher Alasdair MacIntyre sees an ever growing recourse to "emotivism" in modern life, a mode of ethical evaluation that regards all moral judgments as "nothing but expressions of preference, expressions of attitude or feeling."[50] The growing perception that values are unfounded and arbitrary breeds nihilism. Through neglect for their crumbling foundations, it is becoming more difficult to make the case that certain ways of living are more worthwhile than others. Portents of nihilism—nothing matters, anything goes— stir beneath concerns of unease, loss, social decomposition, erosion, and unraveling in modern life. For the scholars we have met in these pages, it is a tragic consequence of the primacy of instrumental reason.

4

IATROGENESIS IN HEALTH PROMOTION

Iatrogenesis is a term of art used to describe the inadvertent harm inflicted by medical practitioners. This chapter presents case studies of the iatrogenic effects of the application of three theories used in designing health promotion interventions: social learning theory, social marketing, and empowerment. The case studies illustrate the ethical pitfalls outlined in the last chapter in concrete terms. The analysis shows how the use of these theories exacerbates, rather than relieves, the dissolution of values underlying so many modern social health problems.

The sociologist and scholar Robert Bellah identifies the flawed starting point from which the field's predicament flows:

> In the social sciences, we study the same kinds of beings we are. Unlike the natural sciences, we are not 'outside' what we study and certainly not 'above' it. To imagine that we are is to deprive those we study of their dignity by treating them as objects. It is also to imagine that we understand them better than they understand themselves because our heads are not filled with the muddled ideas, false consciousness, traditions, and superstitions (murk and vestiges) that theirs are. It is to imagine that we are enlightened and free from illusions. As a result, we are unable to see that we too have our unexamined presuppositions, that we are ourselves involved in promises and commitments, our thoughts and feelings partly molded by symbols we have been given by tradition and do not consciously fully understand.[1]

This chapter examines how a number of the major theories in health promotion are not the value-neutral, objective, scientific accounts proponents believe them to be, but are instead filled with the unexamined presuppositions of the prevailing instrumental mindset of our times.

SOCIAL LEARNING THEORY

Social learning theory (SLT) is arguably the most highly regarded and widely used theory in the field of health promotion today. In a survey of papers published between 1992 and 1994, Glanz, Lewis, and Rimer found that almost one-third of all research reports (148 out of a total of 497 articles) appearing in 24 major health education, medical, and behavioral science journals cited social learning theory or self-efficacy as their theoretical framework. The most frequently referenced theory, SLT, was followed at some distance by the health belief model (100/497) and the theory of reasoned action (66/497).[2] Similarly, in an extensive review of school-based substance abuse programs, William Hansen concluded that social learning theory has demonstrated greater effectiveness in preventing teenage drug use than any other theoretical approach.[3]

In this section, I want to show how social learning theory assumes an utilitarian framework for decision-making, while its proponents present it as an unbiased, scientific explanation of human behavior. Utilitarianism is a theory in moral philosophy that posits that actions should be judged to be right or wrong according to their consequences.[4] The failure to acknowledge the utilitarian underpinnings of SLT is problematic because many philosophers contend that this mode of ethical evaluation distorts sociocultural understandings of the bases for making moral judgments.[5] Because utilitarianism claims all values can be measured on a single scale of quantity of satisfactions, it is antithetical to the idea that values might be qualitatively distinct and incommensurable. Yet Taylor and others argue that qualitative discriminations of worth are essential to the development of moral character and moral responsibility through the exercise of strong second-order evaluation. It is precisely such qualitative distinctions that enable human beings to resolve, with reasoned justifications, that some ways of life are more worthwhile than others, beyond calculations of the amount of pleasure they give. So, when we professionals in the field of health promotion fail to recognize, acknowledge, or challenge the utilitarian foundations of SLT, we may naively and unwittingly participate in promoting a system of thinking that stands opposed to evaluating different courses of action in terms of strong qualitative contrasts: "more or less fulfilling, more or less refined, profound or superficial, virtuous or vicious, courageous or pusillanimous, fragmented or integrated."[6] My concern is that social learning theory is being promulgated in the field as if it were scientifically proven fact, and not as potentially harmful ideology. When researchers and faculty recommend the use of SLT to design programs, I fear that practitioners are not being warned about its utilitarian bias, nor advised that utilitarianism is but one of many different modes of ethical evaluation, nor cautioned that utilitarianism is considered by many to be a significant contributor to the disintegration of values in modern times.

In stating that the sole value of theory resides in its ability to effect change (rather than, say, to contribute to self-knowledge or mutual understanding), Stanford psychologist Professor Albert Bandura, the father of social learning theory, both reflects and reinforces the modern instrumental ethos. Writing in 1977, Bandura's position is unequivocal—the only measure of theory is prediction and control: "Theories must demonstrate predictive power. . . . The value of theory is ultimately judged by the power of the procedures it generates to effect psychological changes."[7] Ten years later, in his most recent book, *Social Foundations of Thought and Action*, he restates his position virtually verbatim: "The value of theory is ultimately judged by its usefulness as evidenced by the power of the methods it yields to effect psychological changes."[8] Conversely, as he makes clear, "Conversation is not an especially effective way of altering human behavior. In order to change, people need corrective learning experiences."[9] As the principal architect of social learning theory, Bandura set out to develop a theory with the power to effectively alter human behavior.

As described by Bandura, SLT is a direct descendent of Skinnerian behaviorism. While behaviorists assert that the individual's thought processes are best regarded as a black box, irrelevant to the task of explaining behavior, social learning theorists put forward a more elaborate model, endowing the individual with a number of cognitive capabilities. They hypothesize that people can observe the behavior of others, remember and anticipate reinforcements, organize them into symbolic codes (verbal or mental representations), and mentally rehearse the behaviors that lead to different reinforcements. The primary difference between SLT and behaviorism is that SLT maintains that people do not have to experience reinforcements directly themselves in order to learn new behaviors; they can also learn through observing what happens to others. Aside from this important modification, social learning theorists accept the basic behaviorist premise that behaviors are governed by reinforcement contingencies. In Bandura's words, "The frequency and durability of a given behavior depends on how the prevailing contingencies of reinforcement are structured."[10]

Despite claims that "Psychology cannot tell people how they ought to live their lives,"[11] Bandura's theory presents one model for thinking about the question of how one ought to live. According to Bandura, the way people make choices is by weighing the costs and benefits—"expectations of positive and negative reinforcements"—of different courses of action: "They fear and avoid things that have been associated with aversive consequences, but like and seek those that have had pleasant associations. They inhibit conduct under circumstances that threaten punishing response consequences, but respond readily in contexts signifying rewardable outcomes."[12] This assertion is a near perfect paraphrase of Jeremy Bentham's original statement of utilitarianism, written in 1789—"Nature has placed mankind under the governance of two sovereign masters, pain and pleasure. It is for them alone to point out what we ought to do, as well as to determine what we shall do"[13]—although Bandura presents it not as a moral principle but as a statement of fact. The calculation of consequences is not presented as a matter of choice among many other possible considerations, but as the determinant of behavior. In Bandura's model, people do not evaluate choices on the basis of a principled understanding of right and wrong, or considerations of duty and obligation, or out of reverent obedience to religious authority, or through reflection upon which ways of life might be more courageous, ennobling, or worthy, but only on the basis of their "pleasant associations" or "aversive consequences." This claim is not put forward as one possible interpretation of human motivation, but as scientifically proven fact. Based on presumptions of scientific objectivity, the classic utilitarian assumptions go unacknowledged.

An example highlights the presumptions of social learning theory and their iatrogenic consequences. Bandura and Taylor have both offered analyses of a common issue and one germane to health promotion, namely, weight control. I cite them at length to let their respective positions speak for themselves.

According to Bandura, "people are motivated to impose upon themselves requirements for self-reward when the behavior they seek to change is aversive. To overweight persons, for example, the discomforts, maladies, and social costs of obesity create inducements to control overeating."[14]

Taylor sees the issue in different terms:

> The utilitarian strand in our civilization would induce us to abandon the language of qualitative contrast, and this means, of course, abandoning strong evaluative languages, for their terms are only defined in contrast. And we can be tempted to redefine issues we are reflecting on in this non-qualitative fashion.
>
> For instance, let us say that I am addicted to overeating. I find it hard to resist treating myself to rich desserts. As I struggle with this issue, in the reflection in which I determine that moderation is better, I can be looking at the alternatives in a language of qualitative contrast. I can be reflecting that someone who has so little control over his appetites that he would let his health go to pot over cream-cake is not an admirable person. I yearn to be free of this addiction, to be the kind of person whose mere bodily appetites respond to his higher aspirations, and don't carry on remorselessly and irresistibly dragging him to incapacity and degradation.
>
> But then I might be induced to see my problem in a quite different light. I might be induced to see it as a question of quantity of satisfaction. Eating too much increases the cholesterol in my blood, makes me fat, ruins my health, prevents me from enjoying all sorts of other desired consumptions; so it isn't worth it. Here I have stepped away from the contrastive language of strong evaluation. Avoiding high cholesterol content, obesity, ill-health, or being able to climb stairs, and so on, can

all be defined quite independently from my eating habits. Someone might even invent some drug which would allow me to go on eating rich desserts and also enjoy all those other goods, whereas no drug would allow me to eat my cake and attain the dignity of an autonomous, self-disciplined agent which I pined after on my first reading of the issue.

It may be that being talked around to seeing things in this non-qualitative light will help me solve my problems, that somehow it was too deeply disturbing when I put it in terms of dignity versus degradation, and now I can come to grips with it. But this is a separate question from deciding which way of putting it is more illuminating and true to reality. This is a question about what our motivation really is, how we should characterize the meaning things have for us. . . .

Let us take the case above of the man who is fighting obesity and who is talked into seeing it as merely a quantitative question of more satisfaction, rather than as a matter of dignity and degradation. As a result of this change, his inner struggle itself becomes transformed, and is now quite a different experience.

The opposed motivations—the craving for cream cake and his dissatisfactions with himself at such indulgence—which are the objects undergoing redescription here, are not independent in the sense outlined above. When he comes to accept the new interpretation of his desire to control himself, the desire itself has altered. True, it may be said on one level to have the same goal, that he stop eating cream cake, but since it is no longer understood as seeking for dignity and self-respect it has become quite a different motivation.[15]

So, the most widely used theory in health education declares that behavior is controlled by reinforcement contingencies. Programs based on SLT are built on this assumption. In order to be effective, participants in health promotion programs designed on the basis of SLT must be talked around into seeing their problem as a matter of rearranging positive and negative reinforcements. The notion that people might be experiencing second-order desires regarding the quality of their appetites in relation to the kind of person they aspire to become does not have a place in this model; the participants need to be persuaded instead to view their motivation in terms of weighing the consequences.[16]

As Taylor's analysis indicates, social learning theory is not a neutral, unbiased explanation of human behavior. It patently assumes a utilitarian framework of human decision-making. When training programs present these theories as scientific truth and health promotion practitioners go on to reproduce these assumptions in program development, they abet those social practices that are undermining our ability to maintain and appreciate distinctions about the quality of our desires, which can only be grasped in terms of strong qualitative contrasts. Over the course of 12 years of teaching these materials, I always ask students to critique the theories presented in class. They have never spontaneously pointed out the utilitarian assumptions underlying SLT, they have difficulty in articulating a forceful critique of utilitarianism, and even more difficulty in laying out alternative modes of ethical reflection. The problem is that these philosophical issues are not covered in standard health promotion textbooks nor research articles, and as a consequence, in failing to address these assumptions, training programs are preparing practitioners to promote an ideology of utility maximization.

SOCIAL MARKETING

Social marketing is a behavioral change model that advocates using commercial marketing principles to influence consumer ideas, attitudes, and lifestyles relating to issues of social concern.[17] The original inspiration for this model is credited to Wiebe, who remarked, "Why can't you sell brotherhood like you sell soap?"[18] Kotler and Zaltman later coined the term "social marketing" in 1971.[19] Andreason defines social marketing as "the application of marketing technologies developed in the commercial sector to the solution of social problems where the bottom line is behavior change."[20] Prominent examples of social marketing campaigns in the United States are "America Responds to AIDS" (ARTA); the privately sponsored "Partnership for a Drug-Free America" (PDFA); and tax-supported antismoking campaigns like those initiated in California and Massachusetts. In 1998, the President and Congress allocated $175 million to a new federal antidrug media campaign designed on social marketing principles.

The increasing use of social marketing creates a number of problems. First, it marks a capitulation to the idea that the ends justify the means. When the ends are thought to justify the means, the integrity of the means is subject to compromise. Then, because of the failure to appreciate the relationship between ends and means in social practices, the use of marketing strategies may result in subverting ends too. In addition, because social practices are not independent of their description, the proliferation of marketing language and assumptions to describe health promotion activities is transforming our self-understanding of our motivations and our relationship to the public in ways inconsistent with the historical values for which the field of health promotion has long stood.

In hiring the Madison Avenue advertising firm, Ogilvy and Mather, to develop the ARTA campaign, the Centers for Disease Control (CDC) has in effect accepted the idea that the ends justify the means. A good case can be made that the primary goal of health promotion is to prevent people from consuming the junk food, cigarettes, and alcohol that advertisers such as Ogilvy and Mather have all too successfully persuaded them to indulge. Similarly, the same corporation, Johnson and Johnson, that markets Valium, Librium, Tylenol-3 with codeine, and numerous other over-the-counter painkillers is the largest corporate sponsor of the Partnership for a Drug-Free America campaign.[21] So, while public health professionals protest the impact of marketing strategies when they are directed toward ends contrary to public health interests, they appear to have few qualms about using the same tactics to achieve the ends they embrace.

Under these circumstances, the means are liable to corruption. The PDFA campaign, for example, has broadcast factually incorrect misinformation from time to time about the consequences of drug use.[22] One of their ads showed an electroencephalogram (EEG) of a person in a coma over the copy, "If you use marijuana, you are not using your brain." Despite appearances, there is no connection between the picture and the text; there are no detectable differences in EEGs between people high on marijuana and those who are not. Likewise, the media tactics of political campaigns frequently fudge the truth to achieve their end. One fears that the equivalent of the notorious Willie Horton ads used in President Bush's bid for reelection will crop up in public health campaigns guided by these principles.

The subversion of means is not limited to misinformation. Richard Pollay, a professor of marketing, has reviewed the work of scholars in the humanities and the social sciences on the social and cultural consequences of advertising.[23] His article summarizes the major themes uncovered in analyses of the processes by which advertising wields its influence. To which human motives does advertising most often make its appeal? Pollay describes the consensus of opinion: "Greed, lust, sloth, and pride were identified earlier [in the article] as common ad themes. One might also consider the extent to which advertising encourages envy and gluttony. If anger were added to the list, we would have what are popularly known as the seven deadly sins."[24] The light tone of his summation should not diminish the gravity of his point. Marketing ads most often pander to the basest of human motives.[25] Are these "communication strategies" appropriate for health promotion?

Not only are the means corrupted, so too the ends. In a brief vignette on the benefits of social marketing, Hastings and Haywood describe their campaign to encourage drinking alcohol in moderation. In their market research, they found that girls think boys who control their drinking are more attractive. The authors state, "This then has implications for the message content of a proposed television advertisement as the 'sexual attractiveness' of drinking in moderation could be promoted as a benefit."[26] Based on a social marketing analysis, they plan to use sex appeal to sell their product, moderate drinking.

Here the methods of social marketing may make us lose sight of the ends of health promotion. There is already widespread concern about the effects of the constant barrage of sexual innuendo in the mass media, especially on young people.[27] Although it is difficult to prove cause and effect, the public in general senses that inundating society with messages framed in terms of sexual attraction is related to the rise of irresponsible sexual behaviors, as evidenced in the ever earlier initiation of sexual activity, rising rates of sexually transmitted diseases (STDs), and the high prevalence of teen pregnancy. The ubiquitous presence of sex in advertising is now an unavoidable part of the socialization process for people growing up in modern society. Hastings and Haywood are suggesting that the use of sex appeals should be extended into one more area of social life.

So, even if this hypothetical campaign were successful in getting young men to drink in moderation, we might not consider it a success if at the same time the campaign promoted sexual promiscuity or denigrated the position of women in society. Not only do the ends not justify the means, but the ends themselves have shifted. We started off wanting people to be healthier, one part of which was thought to be drinking in moderation. But we may end up with moderate drinkers whose images of women as sex objects have been reinforced again.

Pollay continues that many studies have raised concerns that advertising intensifies "materialism, cynicism, irrationality, selfishness, anxiety, social competitiveness, sexual preoccupation, powerlessness, and/or a loss of self-respect."[28] Some of these traits appear already to be creeping into public health promotion campaigns developed using social marketing principles. In several of the new antismoking ads, for example, cigarette manufacturers are portrayed as corrupt evildoers. These ads reinforce societal perceptions that people are generally self-interested, unscrupulous, and watching out only for themselves.[29] This cannot but contribute to the cynicism and mistrust already present in this country.[30]

Finally, the language and ideas of marketing promote one particular understanding of human motivation and human relationships. In their paper, Hastings and Haywood declare, "The concept of exchange is crucial to social marketing."[31] In marketing logic, the "rational" actor is motivated to get the best deal possible for himself and is considered irrational if he fails to maximize the benefits to his self-interests.[32] The exchange relationship between two parties is characterized by this cost–benefit calculus, and if the costs are perceived to be too high, then the parties are expected to go their separate ways. Advocates of social marketing recommend adopting a model of human motivation and human relationships based on this concept of exchange.

Like social learning theory, the central construct of social marketing, the concept of exchange, promotes the idea that people's decisions are motivated by cost–benefit calculations. In developing social marketing campaigns, health promoters are advised to assume that people will opt for health only if the perceived benefits of any proposed behavior change outweigh the perceived costs. Following the lead of advertisers, health promoters are advised to associate non-smoking with a range of perceived benefits, such as sexiness, popularity, and affluence, and to minimize the perceived costs of social rejection or nicotine withdrawal. Once again, if health promoters adopt this model uncritically, I fear its growing use will reinforce the idea that people are fundamentally self-interested utility maximizers, "simple weighers"[33] in Taylor's terms, and move the field farther away from promoting reflection on ends and values beyond the pursuit of self-interests.

For health promotion professionals, as we move increasingly toward adopting marketing terminology to guide our thinking, the concept of exchange should lead us to wonder about what we are getting out of the deal. Health promoters deliver information, skills, and services to the public, for which we should expect to get something from them in exchange. If enough practitioners become convinced to shift into thinking about their work in terms of exchange, then the field may be sapped of a major source of strength. As the balance tips toward expecting quid-pro-quo benefits in exchange for the provision of services, a certain depth of character will become closed off.[34] The increasing penetration of marketing language into all areas of social life displaces and diminishes other frames of reference, specifically the values of altruism, self-sacrifice, and concern for the common welfare.[35]

In contrast to the logic of exchange, people have traditionally entered the health field out of a sense of caring for others, not to maximize self-interests. Most people in public health still feel that to be a health professional means to have a vocation, a sense of calling.[36] They strive to create a healthy society in which no one will be handicapped from participating due to unnecessary illness and suffering. They continue to work in the field out of feelings of sympathy and solidarity with those in need. The yardstick by which their work is measured is the realization of a collective good that flows from the elimination of disease, pollution, hunger, poverty, and oppression. Many of my colleagues have expressed a vague discomfort with the growing enthusiasm for social marketing. At the bottom of these intuitions are concerns about the corruption of means, the deterioration in ends, and the uneasiness that the encroaching use of the language of marketing is warping the terms for thinking about what we are doing and the values for which we stand.

EMPOWERMENT

The final case study concerns the preoccupation with—and problematics of—seeking power to effect social improvement. Interest in obtaining power spans the entire range of interests in the field. In the mainstream scientific camp, power is sought in the form of effective techniques to engineer individual behavioral compliance. Among those in the politically progressive camp, because of the strong association between poverty and the full gamut of health problems, a redistribution of wealth is considered essential to effect improvements in the health of poor and marginalized populations. Progressives thus aim to "empower" oppressed, disenfranchised, and powerless social groups through community organizing techniques in order to bring about this redistribution.[37]

Like most ideas that gain our attention, the concept of power is richly complex and full of ambiguities. Political science, the oldest of the social sciences, has been defined as the study of the shaping and sharing of power. In an engaging exposition of its history, Thomas Wartenberg examines this "essentially contested" [38] concept and maps two main currents: "power over" and "power to." In its classic definition, A is said to have power over B to the extent that A can get B to do what B does not want to do or would not do otherwise.[39] It is the possession of control or command over others, the ability to affect others without their being able to reciprocate, the capacity to produce a change in another person. Power in this sense is synonymous with domination.

Wartenberg traces another stream of thought, the idea of power-as-ability, crediting recent feminist thinking for bringing to light the distinction. "Power to" is the ability to bring about a state of affairs beneficial to the actor. It is possession of the capability to do or effect something, the capacity to produce an intended state of affairs. Power in this sense is equated with liberation and transformation.

This latter definition of power appeals to advocates of empowerment. It appears ethically unproblematic, since it does not have the connotations of domination, coercion, and manipulation. Two questions, however, come to mind: (*1*) whether empowerment strategies can be divorced from these coercive aspects in actual practice, and, (*2*) whether popular interest in empowerment isn't, in fact, more closely related to its traditional definition than proponents care to acknowledge.

Wartenberg draws out a delicate distinction between the two forms of power, citing "relational" versus "nonrelational" uses.[40] "Power over" is concerned with power as it characterizes the relationship between two (or more) people. "Power to" refers to individuals in isolation, as they develop their own capacities independent of interactions with others. But while such a distinction may make sense conceptually, it is not clear to what degree these forms of power are separable in practical terms in the real world. To what extent is it possible to have the "power to" do something without exerting "power over" others? Is it possible to have the "power to" obtain health care, better housing, better education, better transportation, food, childcare, etc., without affecting others, at a minimum getting them to pay more taxes? Are feminists truly not interested in exerting power over men— getting them to do what they do not want or would not do otherwise—who deny them equality in terms of jobs, wages, and household chores? Is it possible to purge the coercive connotations inherent in the traditional understanding of the word and pursue the accumulation of power in a strictly positive, nonrelational sense?

Perhaps. Certainly, there are examples of nonrelational empowerment, such as the "power to" eat less or exercise more, or more broadly, the power to vote or to develop one's creative capacities, such as learning to dance, paint, write poetry, or play a new sport. But more commonly the capacity to produce an intended state of affairs requires resources of some sort, economic or otherwise. It takes real material resources to accomplish much in this world, which leads back to an interest in power in its classic form, getting people to do that which they would not do otherwise, like pay taxes. Ironically, for a field dependent on public financing, when advocates claim they are interested in power only in its ethically unproblematic, nonrelational sense, they align themselves with conservative politicians like Jack Kemp who invoke the language of empowerment in order to deny the need for government support.

The ambiguities inherent in the concept of power have carried over to its use in health promotion. In a recent unprecedented two-volume special issue of *Health Education Quarterly*, virtually all the researchers introduce their articles by duly noting the "lack of clarity about the conceptualization of empowerment" and the "widely varying definitions and assumptions" behind its use.[41] They then generally proceed to gloss over these ambiguities or treat them as if they could be exorcised through definitional fiat. The question is whether the enthusiasm for empowerment raises any issues about which we should be concerned.

To begin, it might be worth pausing to ask, "Why empowerment?" "Why has empowerment assumed such prominence in the field these days?" Of all the different candidates that could possibly be contemplated, why has the interest in power become so predominant? Why not caring, or compassion, or dignity, or love, morality, respect, harmony, responsibility, or some other significant human aspiration? Why has the pursuit of power captured so much attention?

As Gitlan reminds us, people think within the intellectual and cultural currents that surround them, currents with histories even if their sources cannot be seen from downstream.[42] Weber's concerns about the rise of instrumental reason and the subsequent crumbling foundations of values are deeply indebted to one of his contemporaries. To understand the current interest in power and to see the full dimensions of the modern predicament, it may be worthwhile to retrace this intellectual current back to its original source. The prophetic German philosopher Friedrich Nietzsche was the first to call attention to the will to power.

Writing during the late 1890s and early 1900s, Nietzsche implores in one of his more celebrated passages:

> Have you not heard of that madman who, in the broad light of forenoon, lit a lantern, and ran into the marketplace, crying incessantly: "I am looking for God!" . . . As it happened, many were standing there who did not believe in God, and so he aroused great laughter. . . . The madman leapt right among them. . . . "Where is God?" he cried. "Well, I will tell you. We have murdered him—you and I. But how did we do this deed? . . . Who gave us the sponge with which to wipe out the whole horizon? How did we set about unchaining our earth from her sun? Whither is it moving now? Whither are we moving? . . . Are we not falling incessantly? . . . Is not night approaching, and more and more night? Must we not light lanterns in the forenoon? Behold the noise of the gravediggers, busy to bury God. . . . And we have killed him! What possible comfort is there for us? . . . Is not the greatness of this deed too great for us? To appear worthy of it, must not we ourselves become gods?"—At this point the madman fell silent and looked once more at those around him: "Oh," he said, "I am too early. My time is not yet come. The news of this tremendous event is still on its way. . . . Lightning and thunder take time, the light of the stars takes time to get to

us, deeds take time to be seen and heard . . . and *this* deed is still farther from them than the farthest stars—*and yet it was they themselves who did it!*"[43]

Writing 300 years after Sir Francis Bacon laid the foundations of modern thought, Nietzsche was deeply disturbed by the perception that the premodern metaphysic was crumbling—the belief that the cosmos was meaningful and infused with an ordained set of God-given values, which it was man's purpose to fathom in finding his rightful place in the cosmological order. So long as human beings saw themselves a divine creation, the evaluation of human actions could be firmly secured with reference to divine intentions. The basis for judging the quality of lives was the extent to which they fulfilled the purposes of their Creator.

But modernity heralded the death of God, which for Nietzsche was both a cultural and a philosophical event: the evident decline of Christianity and the abandonment of metaphysics as such, transcendent systems of thought contemplating the meaning of human existence. "One interpretation of existence has been overthrown," he exclaimed, "but since it was held to be *the* interpretation, it seems as though there were no meaning in existence at all, as though everything were in vain."[44] In the wake of the God's death, Nietzsche was profoundly troubled by what he saw as the aftermath: an ensuing state of nihilism, the obliteration of all distinctions in value. "People have no notion yet that from now onwards they exist on a mere pittance of inherited and decaying values. . . . I foresee something terrible, Chaos everywhere. Nothing left which is of any value; nothing which commands: Thou shalt!"[45]

Nietzsche beheld traditional religious ways of thinking on the wane, leaving a void science could not fill. Contrary to common misperceptions, his lifework did not extol nihilism but was feverishly consumed with trying to overcome it, in conceiving how to generate the revaluation of values. How should humanity respond as they gradually come to realize they have to accept responsibility for giving meaning to their own existence?[46]

Into this void—in a way that he was never able to work out satisfactorily before his collapse—he injected the notion of the Will to Power. Zarathustra's mission was to lead men away from myth and toward the will to power. "What is good?—All that heightens the feeling of power, the will to power, power itself in man. What is bad?—All that is born of weakness. What is happiness?—The feeling that power increases—that a resistance is overcome. Not contentment but more power; *not* peace at all, but war; not virtue but proficiency."[47]

The surviving notes and fragments of Nietzsche's final work in progress, *The Will To Power*, are subject to many interpretations. At points, he seems to treat the will to power as the most basic motivation of human life, and indeed, all living things; at points, it seems the will to power is used as a generic definition of morality. While it would be remiss to conclude he meant the will to power as the ultimate solution to the revaluation of values, that is how many people have read his thinking. The will to power should replace reason. Might makes right. Many have come finally to accept the ancient counsel, "Justice is nothing but the will of the stronger."

Bereft of absolutes, if there is no reasoned basis for adjudicating value claims, the siren call of wielding power to enforce claims becomes ever more seductive. Buffeted by these same currents of thought, the field of health promotion struggles to find solid ground. Instead of exercising practical reason, the field turns to the methodological proficiency of instrumental reason. Instead of research seeking clarity about the good life for human beings, the field seeks certainty about the most effective and efficient means to effect change in others' behaviors. Instead of mutual deliberation in civil society, the field seeks to empower groups so that their definition of justice will prevail. The interest in power is not a coincidence; it suits the temper of the times.

The field of health promotion has joined the bandwagon of empowerment wholeheartedly, leaving its dark side unannounced and unexplored. The mainstream scientific view, with its resources committed to finding the power to control the behavior of others, calls for "voluntary participation" to wash its hands of the intent to manipulate. More liberal advocates of empowerment wish to see themselves as promoting only the positive sense of power as ability, begging the question of whether one person's gain is another person's loss.

Only the old communists and their fellow travelers acknowledge they are after power in its traditional sense, militantly lining up to overthrow the historical forces of oppression—capitalism, racism, sexism, etc. While there is little evidence of things going to this extreme these days, it is this same impulse that animated leftists and black power activists to stockpile weapons in the sixties. They have a point (although there are ironies here too, as we shall see later).[48] There is no question that campaign contributors and lobbyists wield enormous power to benefit the rich, promote corporate interests, and extend inequality. Yet how should we respond? Liberal appeals for progressive taxation and a redistribution in wealth have thus far been unable to make the case—to offer a compelling enough vision of a better world that the majority of people would choose to contribute their resources to secure the growth of the common good. Marx never worked out how life would look after the revolution.

In conclusion, my concern is that the push for empowerment teaches that exerting power is the best way to get what one wants. When health promotion specialists advocate and disseminate empowerment strategies, there is a corresponding depreciation of the value of reason, dialogue, and deliberation. The preference given empowerment breeds cynicism. People cannot be reasoned with—one must muster powerful tactics to make them do one's bidding. Talk of empowerment is de rigeur in Holyoke. The value of education and the possibility of reaching reasoned agreement are not getting equal time.

But there is no denying my friends' protests. At some point, people lose patience with talk. For how many more years will we continue to tolerate poverty, unemployment, and homelessness, and continue to let the burden fall disproportionately on people of color? For all my talk about free will and the individual's capacity for choosing different courses of action based on different conceptions of the kinds of lives most worth living, what kind of choices do people without jobs, without food, without homes have? Who should be held responsible in situations where people make bad choices because those are the only ones they have? People turn to desperate measures when they see no signs or hope of progress.

Engaging community members in deliberations about our collective responsibility for curing these ills is the most important task for the field. While I sympathize with those who believe exercising power is the only way we will make things better, I want to hold out another possibility. With a better idea of the pitfalls of the direction in which we are now headed, it is time to turn to a discussion of a positive alternative. Instead of the will to power, the second half of the book recommends the exercise of practical reason in civil society to promote individual and community well-being.

5

PRACTICAL REASON

The distinction between practical reasoning and scientific reasoning, while well-established in philosophical circles, is virtually unknown among health researchers. The idea that the process of getting answers to questions about what ought to be done in the sociopolitical domain—derived from judgment, deliberation, and wisdom—is different from the process of getting answers to questions about the nature of relationships between objects in the natural world, has a long history.[1] But this difference has never been seriously considered in public health promotion and, in the perennial discussions about the gap between theory and practice, practitioners find themselves constantly on the defensive for not demonstrating stronger scientific foundations for their efforts. This chapter describes practical reason and explains why it is a more viable and more coherent intellectual frame of mind for guiding the practice of public health promotion. In these pages, public health promoters will see that practical reason is an essential and quotidian part of their work. Let me give an example.

New data have just come out showing that Holyoke has the second highest rate of infant mortality in Massachusetts, after rising for 3 years in a row. We would like to mobilize a community response but do not want to provoke an over-reaction, or outbursts of anger and finger-pointing blame. The numbers are small and need to be presented judiciously. With a history of strained community relations, Director Ernie Mathieu fears the health department will be denounced for not having done more, when in fact they have no resources to address infant mortality. What should we do? A new mayor has recently been elected and seems to be more supportive of health and human service programs than the previous administration. But he is sensitive to a conservative constituency and wonders aloud about whether the data might be seen as further evidence of the waste of government programs. When we meet with him, he makes passing reference to "those people," referring to the Puerto Rican community. It sounds vaguely racist, but I am not sure. Should I call him on it? What good would that do? Do I have the guts to do it? Or should I bite my tongue, in the hope that he will become engaged in the issue and learn from the experience? After years of neglect, the leader of a local teen pregnancy coalition resents the new-found official interest in the issue and is initially antagonistic toward entreaties to join forces. The coordinator of the Latino community coalition is a young, bright activist but flamboyant in dress and demeanor, not the kind of community leader the mayor wants representing his official response. How do we proceed? What can I say that will help all the parties involved see more clearly the good that could come from working together? How can I listen well to hear and be swayed by their conflicting visions of the best way to proceed? I discuss my concerns with a mentor, the head of the regional office of the Department of Public Health. "It's politics," she remarks. "You know, everything they never teach you in school."

With this small taste of the exercise of practical reason, the chapter opens with several definitions of practical reason. It then highlights three characteristic differences between practical reason and instrumental scientific reasoning. This is followed by numerous everyday applied examples of the use of practical reason in health promotion. The chapter concludes with a response to positivist questions about the validity of practical reason.

DEFINITION AND CHARACTERISTICS

Aristotle is credited with making the original distinction between scientific and practical reason, based on the distinct categories of human experience he termed *theoria* and *praxis*. Anthony Kenny explains Aristotle's distinction:

> Practical reasoning is reasoning which reasons out the good, as theoretical reasoning is reasoning which reasons out the truth. The conclusion of a piece of theoretical reasoning is a truth to be believed; the conclusion of a piece of practical reasoning is a good to be brought about. By setting out my theoretical reasoning I may explain why I believe a certain proposition; by setting out my practical reasoning I may explain why I am performing a certain action. . . . The point of practical reasoning is the achievement of good, just as the point of theoretical reasoning is the acquisition of truth.

The most important difference between the two kinds of reasoning can be stated as follows. If a theoretical proposition is true, then it cannot conflict with any other theoretical proposition. But sound practical premises may conflict with each other; that is to say, a premise expressing the goodness of a certain value or course of action may very well conflict with another premise expressing the goodness of a different value or incompatible course of action.[2]

The political scientist Peter Steinberger defines the differences this way. "We recognize there is often a very great difference between being wise and being knowledgeable. . . . *Phronesis* [practical reason] is concerned entirely with the intrinsic merits of actions (*praxis*). The scientist or mathematician is forced, so to speak, by the true and ineluctable features of the world to believe this or that proposition. . . . This means, among other things, that the conclusion of any scientific argument is strictly determined by the unchanging facts of the world. Things are as they are and cannot be otherwise. . . . *Phronesis*, on the other hand, is a matter of choice. It is involved in rendering judgments, making decisions, and performing actions that, as Aristotle would have it, 'could have been other than they are.'"[3]

Stuart Hampshire emphasizes the point that practical reason addresses normative questions; it is the thought process involved in reflecting on what one ought to do. "A person asks himself, or is asked by another, a normative question about an activity in which he is engaged: 'Why do you think you should do this?' . . . In the *Nichomachean Ethics*, Aristotle represents the process of brooding on the proper target of one's conduct as the first and fundamental form of practical reasoning."[4] Continuing elsewhere, Hampshire writes, "Aristotle recognized that deliberation about practical possibilities ('What should I do?' 'What is the right thing to do in these circumstances?') is the primary form of moral thought from which the primary form of moral judgment emerges: the judgment that of all the possibilities that are open, the best action to take, all things considered, is so-and-so."[5]

With these definitions in mind, I would like to highlight three contrasts between practical and scientific reasoning. These are by no means exhaustive, but they bring out the major critical differences. First, practical reasoning focuses on the ends of action; the primary object of attention in practical reasoning is the good, the aims, and purposes of action (in contrast to instrumental reason, where the focus is on the means). Second, the criteria for determining the "goodness" of choice cannot be specified in advance in matters of practical reason, but rather good judgment is based on discernment and insight into the singularly salient features of the particular situation at hand. In contrast, in seeking answers to questions through the scientific method, formal procedural criteria are established *a priori* (i.e., random assignment, *p*-values, etc.). Third, practical reason views means and ends as inextricably intertwined, rather than as separate and independent issues.

Reflection on Ends

Practical reason distinguishes itself from instrumental reason first and foremost through its characteristic reflection on the ends, or *telos*, of action. Practical reason is centrally concerned with clarifying goals and deciding which goals are most worthwhile. It is the thought process we use when we consciously ponder questions about the good we are trying to bring about in situations requiring action. In everyday settings, people pause to ask themselves, "What should we do?" Practical reason is the faculty of judgment that answers such questions.

The philosopher Hans Georg Gadamer emphasizes the point, "What separates [practical reason] fundamentally from technical expertise is that it expressly asks the question of the good too—for example, about the best way of life or the best constitution of the state. It does not merely master an ability."[6] Unlike instrumental reason, practical reason focuses on thinking about the value of all the diverse ends that could possibly be achieved in the situation at hand and thinking about which course is best in light of the various potential good outcomes.[7]

Practical reason evaluates and reevaluates goals. The reader may recall Selznick's words: "Moral reason . . . makes goals problematic and broadens responsibilities. It asks: Are the postulated goals worth pursuing in light of the means they seem to require? Are the institution's values, as presently formulated, worthy of realization? What costs are imposed on *other* ends and *other* values?"[8] In health promotion, we engage this faculty of judgment when we ask questions about the goals we are trying to achieve. What do we mean by human well-being? Is biological fitness the ideal, the highest goal of the field? Is biological fitness worth pursuing if it means we must employ technologies to modify behavior and effectively enforce compliance with prescribed regimens of diet and exercise? What are the costs of such manipulation in relation to other ends and other values, such as autonomy, responsibility, and respect for the dignity and integrity of individual community members? In contrast to an instrumental mindset, greater recognition, legitimation, and use of practical reason would mean that health promotion specialists would enter situations open to the possibility that, in the exchange of views with community members, they may have occasion to rethink and revise the goals they are seeking.

Criteria of Choice

The fact that there are different foci of attention for practical and instrumental reason has major implications for what is considered relevant for making determinations. In scientific reasoning, determinations of the validity of an empirical proposition (is this true?) are made through rigorous adherence to the scientific method. In practical reasoning, determinations of the validity of normative propositions (is this good?) are made through sensitive perception of the unique possibilities for realizing the substantive values pregnant in each situation. In scientific reasoning, a priori formal procedural criteria are used to answer research questions. In practical reason, it is the good itself (the goals, ends, purposes) that is under question and determinations of the most worthwhile course of action are made through being open to the *gestalt* of the situation, through being sensitive, attentive, and mindful of all relevant elements and mutual moral relationships in the situation at hand. The quality of decisions is directly related to the quality of perceptions, through attention to detail, nuance, and fine distinctions. Succinctly stated, "*Phronesis* or practical reason involves an irreducible element of perception of the particular, that just here and now, this is the right thing to do."[9]

Martha Nussbaum elaborates the point. Because of the mutability, indeterminancy, and particularity of social situations, practical reason involves:

> the ability to discern, acutely and responsively, the salient features of one's particular situation. The Aristotelian conception argues that this ability is at the core of what practical wisdom is. . . . For he makes it clear that it is in the very nature of truly rational practical choice that it cannot be made more 'scientific' without becoming worse. Instead, he tells us, the 'discernment' of the correct choice rests with something that he calls 'perception.' From the context it is evident that this is some sort of complex responsiveness to the salient features of one's concrete situation.
>
> Aristotle's position is subtle and compelling. It seems to me to go further than any other account of practical rationality I know in capturing the sheer complexity and agonizing difficulty of choosing well. . . . He explicitly claims that priority in practical choice should be accorded not to principle, but to perception, a faculty of discrimination that is concerned with apprehending concrete particulars. . . . The subtleties of a complex ethical situation must be seized in a confrontation with the situation itself, by a faculty that is suited to address it as a complex whole. Prior general formulations lack both the concreteness and the flexibility that is required. . . . Aristotle argues for the ethical priority of concrete description to general statement, particular judgment to general rule.[10]

Hence, for Aristotle, one of the most crucial characteristics of practical reason is that "The decision lies with the perception."[11]

As the complexity of responding to the infant mortality data in Holyoke suggests, the sorts of arguments one ought to use to elicit people's cooperation cannot be specified in advance. The history, cast of characters, and their relationships are never going to be exactly the same in Omaha, Seattle, or anywhere else. Practical choices cannot be made through reference to scientific theories, which are formulated by identifying the most generalizable features, because one must tailor one's choice to the complex requirements of the concrete situation at hand. To choose well, one needs to pick up the easily missed and unforeseeable features there and then, to be open to new impressions, and to be receptive to unexpected inputs, that may change one's judgment. Practical reasoning is the ability to read a situation and single out the most relevant features.

The different criteria for making determinations arise because of fundamental ontological differences in their respective domains. As Kenny noted, scientific facts cannot contradict one another (e.g., increasing the temperature cannot both increase the pressure and decrease the pressure). But claims about the validity and goodness of different values can, and often do, conflict with one another. Because of these differences, the application of scientific method is ill-suited for making practical determinations. In the sociopolitical domain, we need to employ a different reasoning process as we try to balance conflicting values and determine the right course of action.

In the social sphere, we frequently find ourselves in situations with conflicting moral demands, for example, conflicts between truth and kindness, or fairness and friendship. You make a promise to finish a project by a certain time, but your mother's deteriorating health requires more attention than anticipated. In these situations, the application of any sort of means–ends calculus is irrelevant because it is the end itself that is in question—which one is more important. In these situations, the choice one makes depends on one's reading of the situation. These choices, in turn, define the kind of person we become.

In the social world, choices may differ from person to person and yet both can be good choices. Kenny explains, "Wisdom will prescribe differently in the two cases because of the different overarching end which constitutes the chief happiness of each of the two types of virtuous persons."[12] Individuals make choices in light of their own projects and aims, which give the situation its particular meaning for that person. Practical deliberation is concerned with questions about whether a certain course of action will move the agent toward realizing some important value that constitutes the kind of person one strives to be and without which one's life would be less valuable. Should I challenge the mayor about his vaguely racist reference? I can make one choice—and another person the opposite choice—and we can still understand them both to be good choices. Both can be the right thing to do under those circumstances based on each person's understanding of his or her larger purposes in life.[13]

The claim that decisions should be based on perceptions of the particular situation has led critics to protest that this outlook recommends nothing more than situational, and therefore, unprincipled, ethics.[14] Nussbaum responds that decisions that value the keen perception of particular contexts and hold this to be criterial of good choice need not in any sense be relativistic.[15] In the situation above, when someone has made a promise, yet also feels obligated to care for her mother, what is the overriding principle that should be invoked? A person of practical wisdom is a person of integrity with a highly developed understanding of principles of justice, equality, inclusion, truthfulness, and positive freedom, yet who still may be faced with the necessity of making a choice between irresolvably conflicting value demands. The choice will be based on the particular circumstances, but that does not in any way make it unprincipled, arbitrary, or relativistic.

Finally, practical reason is not deductive, it is more like sense perception. Where scientific reason relies on deductive methods (testing hypotheses derived from abstract theories), practical reason is casuistic.[16] Practical reason looks to case studies to reveal the broadest range of potential considerations that may have a bearing on the situation at hand. Practical deliberations are made better through knowledge of actual cases, detailed examples of deliberations, choices, and their attendant consequences, historical accounts, analogies, and the like, that illustrate subtle discriminations between good and bad choices. One familiar way to grasp the distinction here is by thinking about the respective processes through which we assess the quality of literature versus the way we conduct experiments. Regarding the former, there is no set of steps that one can or must follow to decide what commends a good book.[17] In the latter case, there are procedures that one must follow in order to draw sound conclusions in answer to research questions. Steinberger likens the process of exercising and improving one's judgment to the process of gaining an ear for music, of being able to hear when the tempo or phrasing on Rachmaninoff's Piano Concerto #3 is not right. "It is an activity that proceeds in ways that cannot be reduced to the standard methods of science, that operates not at all in terms of fixed and defensible rules or algorithms."[18]

Because there are no set procedures to follow, Aristotle thought there was no substitute for experience in improving people's capacity for exercising good judgment. Citing Aristotle's original distinction, Larmore notes, "No one can acquire judgment by being imparted some formal doctrine. It can only be learned through practice, through being trained in the performance of right actions."[19]

Relationship between Means and Ends

To introduce the concept of a virtue at this point, the philosopher Alisdair MacIntyre identifies the core difference between natural processes and social practices, and hence, the different relationships between means and ends:

> When we speak of any happening or state or activity as a means to some other, we mean that the world is as a matter of contingent fact so ordered that if you are able to bring about a happening or state or activity of the first kind, an event or state or activity of the second kind will ensue. The means and the end can each be adequately characterized without reference to one another; and a number of quite different means may be employed to achieve one and the same end. But the exercise of the virtues is not in this sense *a* means to the end of the good for man. For what constitutes the good for man is a complete human life lived at its best, and the exercise of the virtues is a necessary and central part of such a life, not merely a preparatory exercise to secure such a life. We thus cannot characterize the good for man adequately without already having made reference to the virtues.[20]

The differences between instrumental and practical reason emerge due to essential differences between the natural and social worlds. In the natural world, the relationship between means and ends is independent in two senses of the word. First, the effect that results from a given cause is independent of the observer's characterization of the outcome. Scientists are forced, so to speak, by the ineluctable features of the natural world to accept that the effect of increasing the current in electrical circuits is to increase the volts, or potential electromotive force, when the resistance remains constant ($E = ir$). This is a fact, it is the way the world is, and researchers have no choice in the matter. Second, a given effect can be produced independently through changing any number of (independent) causes. Increasing the current increases the voltage; likewise, increasing the resistance increases the voltage. Either means can be used to produce the same result.

In the social world, the relationship between means and ends is not independent, in both senses. The effect that results is not independent from the observer's characterization of the outcome. That is, the good that results is a matter of interpretation; it is not something that is given by the structure of the universe. Abortion is an effective means of birth control, but there is widespread disagreement about whether the outcome is good or not. Second, the effect is not independent of the means used to produce it. Rather, the quality of outcomes is shaped in large measure by the means used to achieve them. There is no moral equivalence between the prevention of teen pregnancy by forcing every female to accept Norplant implants at puberty and the prevention of teen pregnancy by teenagers' exercising their free choice to remain abstinent. The results are not the same because the means used are an intrinsic part of how we characterize the outcomes in the social domain. We get ourselves into trouble when we apply scientific thinking to events in the social world. In the social world, the quality or goodness of an outcome depends on the means used to achieve it.[21]

Now we have a better context for understanding Bellah's observation cited earlier, "It is precisely the point about *praxis* that it has no extraneous product. It has an end, namely, the good of human beings, but that end is attained through itself, that is, through action or practice that is ethical and political. . . . The purpose is not to produce or to control anything but to discover through mutual discussion and reflection between free citizens the most appropriate ways, under present conditions, of living the ethically good life. For 'helping professionals, this would involve toleration of high levels of uncertainty in trying to aid people to improve their own skills of practical autonomy, rather than categorizing them in terms of preconceived theories with resulting automatic formulas for treatment."[22]

This short summary of key differentiating characteristics between scientific and practical reason may prompt two wildly contrary reactions: nonchalant acceptance or appalled aversion. On the former, some people may respond that the allegedly distinctive characteristics of practical reason are not really new or different: the idea of tailoring responses to the particulars of a given situation is a well-accepted principle in the field. In *Health Behavior and Health Education*, Glanz and her colleagues declare, "He or she [the professional] does not blindly follow a cookbook recipe but constantly creates the recipe anew, depending on the circumstances."[23]

It is hard to know what to make of this statement. The authors are strong, unequivocal advocates for the positivist experimental scientific foundations of health education, yet they rather incongruently recommend abandoning central tenets of this system of thought. As researchers, Glanz, Lewis, and Rimer would hardly tolerate the idea of field staff creating anew, depending on the site, their own measures of the independent and dependent variables under investigation. Likewise, they would scoff at any physicist who claimed to have discovered "cold fusion" but announced that other scientists would not necessarily have to follow the reportedly successful procedures identically. They know it would be irresponsible for a chemist producing zidovudine (AZT) to make up his own formula for its manufacture, instead of assiduously conforming to the exact methods for its production each time. They know full well that it is patients who have not adhered to prescribed drug regimens that have given rise to drug-resistant tuberculosis. The incongruity, I think, is a tacit admission of the disparity between the requirements for good practice in health promotion and the standards of science. While they may let slip the need for creativity depending on the circumstances, it is not consistent with the commitment to the positivist paradigm.

The latter reaction—swift rejection—arises because many people seem to fear that any move away from the field's scientific foundations would open the floodgates to a slew of capricious nonsense, with no tools left to distinguish fact from fiction, truth from fantasy. The great appeal of scientific reasoning is that it provides definitive criteria for accepting or rejecting claims (e.g., $p < 0.05$). Practical reason appears to offer no such comparable, clear-cut criteria for determining the validity of any statement. Before turning to questions about how we know that a given judgment is correct, I would like to present a number of examples of the everyday use of practical reason in health promotion to set the stage for a discussion of its warrants and validity.

THE PRIORITY OF PRACTICAL REASON

Imagine a week in the life of the average health promotion specialist. It is filled with attending meetings, conducting workshops and trainings, leading discussions, producing educational materials, preparing reports, meeting with city officials, preparing press releases, initiating and participating in community coalitions, setting priorities, collaborating with personnel from other agencies, and responding to a welter of requests. My contention is that scientific knowledge offers little help for health promotion specialists to do their jobs well. On the contrary, almost all of their actions require the exercise of practical reason.

In my experience, a tremendous amount of time in public health promotion is spent in meetings. A group of people meets to figure out what to do about a particular problem. They start by trying to figure out what the problem is exactly and what their goals should be, weighing different possibilities. The health promoter sits there listening, pondering whether and when to speak out and when to rest content during the course of the conversation. Carefully attending to the exchanges, she considers whether someone has mischaracterized an element of the problem, misrepresented the efforts of a particular person or agency, or missed an important point and whether she needs to point out these oversights. She mulls over how she can frame her remarks so they will be taken well. On reflection, she thinks the discussion appears to be headed in the right direction—sure, there may be a few minor points to quibble about, but on the whole the group's deliberations are on the right track. Interrupting to raise minor concerns would be distracting and would not be making a worthwhile contribution. Now the discussion seems stuck, the group is not sure where they are. She has an inspiration, an insight that may move people past this sticking point, and speaks up. One begins to get a picture of the process of practical reasoning.

Health promoters are frequently called upon to facilitate meetings. How does one decide which items to put on the agenda, how much time they will require, and which issues will have to wait until a later meeting? After struggling to put together an agenda, the most common experience once the meeting starts is that the facilitator must continually grapple with judgments about letting a discussion run on one point or cutting it off to move onto other business. Has the discussion become sidetracked, drifting off on an interesting yet incidental tangent? Is this unanticipated discussion important enough, or does the group need to get back to the original agenda? How does the facilitator decide if the current discussion is more valuable than other business, or at least valuable enough? At what point does he say something to let people know why he has decided to let the dialogue continue? Or should he, and how should he, interrupt to press forward with the agenda? Or should he let the group decide? The facilitator then tries to summarize the discussion and the consensus of group opinion. Choosing his words well, as opposed to saying something that shows he was inattentive, insensitive, and missed a subtle point, makes the difference between running a successful meeting and frustrating or confusing people, leaving them wondering what, if any, decisions were made.

In similar fashion, writing up the minutes to a meeting is an art. Capturing the gist of a discussion is difficult. More often than not, discussions are rambling, interspliced with several different points at once, never quite finishing up one discussion before someone brings up something else, only to return to the original point later in the meeting. How does one weave the various threads together? A good set of minutes can give the group a sense of progress; incoherent jottings (which may more closely resemble verbatim transcripts) leave everyone bewildered, forcing people to go back over the same ground at the next meeting. In addition, discussions frequently touch upon sensitive issues, such as the reputation of an agency or person. How these comments are recorded and presented requires tact, discretion. These judgments also depend on the audience receiving copies of the minutes. Where is the theory here?

New data show the local community to have the highest infant mortality rate in the state. Perhaps the health promoter has been formally trained in public health and ponders whether to propose the more militant, confrontational strategy defined by community organization theory, or the more consensual, "bottom up" approach described by community development theory. How does the practitioner decide? A good practitioner will base her decision on her knowledge of the history of the community, the demographic composition of the community, the players and personalities involved, their history of working together, how infant mortality relates to other issues in the community, the likelihood of cooperation or resistance from various different stakeholders, her reputation and experience in the community, and a host of other considerations. As a brief perusal of the list suggests, there is no formula—no equivalent of calculating the sample size to attain a certain degree of statistical power—that is going to determine what she should do. Everything depends on a sensitive, perceptive assessment of the local situation, its unique features, and the specific context. Her decision requires perspicacious judgment.

Say she reflects on the issue and decides the time is ripe for a new spirit of collaboration. She recommends using community development theory. What should she say to convince others who feel less sanguine about the prospects for cooperation and are advocating instead more aggressive tactics, such as sit-ins, pickets, and demonstrations to demand new programs, as specified in community organizing theory? Suppose she rallies her wits and her view prevails. Is she now in a position to go about manipulating a set of identified independent variables? No. Typically, the practitioner will have to find the right balance between exerting her own leadership on the issue and fostering community ownership. When should she stand up, take a strong position at meetings, and when should she let others take charge, even if initial steps appear somewhat plodding? Finding the right balance will depend on her remaining attuned to the ebb and flow of a complicated situation with all its distinct characteristics.

She meets with the mayor to seek his support with this new initiative. She knows he is Catholic and considers whether this might be a worthwhile way to relate and connect with one another and press the importance of the issue. It may or may not be appropriate depending on many circumstances: whether she is Catholic too, whether they attend the same church, what their respective ages are, whether they attended the same parochial school, and how upfront each of them is about their religious faith. During the course of their meeting, he says something that sounds vaguely racist. Now she is reporting back on her meeting with the mayor to the larger group. How does she characterize their meeting? What is the good she is seeking to realize? It all depends on the particulars of the situation: who she is and her experiences with racism; who the mayor is (black? white? Asian?), what is known about his history, and where he has stood on the issue; the history of their personal and professional relationships; her assessment of the specific composition of the larger group and how they might react; her assessment of whether his remarks were sufficiently harsh such that she has had to reassess her own position about the prospects for cooperation; and so on. A rash appraisal would likely precipitate a mess of unwanted outcomes.

The group decides to hold a press conference and she agrees to write the press release. She is concerned that the local media may portray infant mortality as a racial issue, reinforce stereotypes, and aggravate community tensions. She agonizes over how to frame the data so that all segments of the community will feel they have a stake in the issue. She thinks about who should be the spokesperson for the group at the press conference. She weighs the tradeoffs between someone who may be more articulate and comfortable in front of the press versus someone who is more representative of the community. What is the right answer? At the press conference, a reporter asks an unexpected and complicated question: "What is the group's position on distributing birth control devices in school clinics?" Under the glare of klieg lights, how should the spokesperson respond? She pauses to consider whether she knows the reporter and his position on the issue, the paper he works for, and how much she can trust his representation of her remarks. Is he sincere, or is he fishing for a sensationalistic hook for a storyline? Should she answer directly, stonewall the question, or deflect it with humor? It was precisely Aristotle's point that science will never be able to calculate the most effective response in situations like these.

The group wants to invite more people to join the effort. How do they decide whom to invite? How about local businesses? the Knights of Columbus? the Parent Teacher Organization (PTO)? What do they do about agencies that have a history of mutual antagonism? How do they approach working with the local teen pregnancy coalition leader, who thinks she should be in charge, yet has managed over the years to alienate several critical groups from participating in her coalition? The next meeting is called, but some person or some group is overlooked—and outraged. How does one mend fences? In the exercise of practical reason, Nussbaum replies, "The only way to proceed here is to put oneself on the line with as much sincerity and accuracy as possible, showing what it takes to be truly deep and pertinent."[24]

The health promoter is invited out to the local high school to conduct a workshop on substance abuse. She wants to use the most effective intervention possible and so pulls out a prepackaged curriculum. It is distributed by a private corporation marketing the work of unknown authors with impressive-looking credentials. The curriculum seems to be based on Social Learning Theory—there is frequent mention of positive reinforcements—but it is not explicitly stated. She reviews the materials and prepares for the trainings. But when she arrives, she senses something is wrong; it feels like the students are upset. She stops, asks, and learns the students have not volunteered to attend. They are fed up with hearing about drugs and feel like their needs and concerns are being ignored. What should she do? Do the students have a right to decide what they think is most important to discuss? Are the goals of the meeting up for discussion?

You have just shown a film on sex education and are leading the discussion. A student raises a question, and, at first glance, you are puzzled by the question. You do not see the connection to the day's topic. Do you politely ignore the question and move on with the discussion? Or do you take time to find out what he is going on about, to try to work with him to articulate more clearly his fuzzy understanding of the relevance of his concerns?

I am meeting with a group of residents to talk about the high rates of substance abuse and AIDS in the community. They interrupt my presentation and begin to ask me personal questions, asking me about my history and experiences with drugs and unsafe sexual encounters. I sense they are testing the waters, that they are trying to figure out how much they can trust me, how open we can be, how much we can connect and relate to one another. So what should I do? Go on with the presentation, maintaining a detached professional demeanor? Or do I acknowledge that I share the same struggles they do, that I do not have privileged professional access to arcane scientific knowledge regarding the causes that push people to make bad choices, and that I do not have some special technique for changing my life or theirs?

The health promoter is preparing for a meeting with the City Council to discuss the health department's budget for next year. She is poring over a ton of health statistics and trying to decide what to include in her presentation. What is the overall tone she is trying to set? Should she emphasize areas of progress, where the health department is succeeding, or call attention to problem areas, where more needs to be done? How much information should she try to present? At what point does it become overwhelming, a numbing blur of disembodied numbers? How much should she stress the human side and how much the "hard data?" How technical should the report be? Should she include relative risk ratios with their associated confidence intervals? The answers to these questions depend on a sensitive perception of the particular situation: what has happened in years past; are the city councilors supportive or antagonistic toward the health department; do any of the city councilors have a health background; is the city budget going up or going down; is the city's population more liberal or more conservative; what else is going on locally at that time.

You spend 3 months collecting a wealth of information from various community groups about their recommendations concerning AIDS. How do you prioritize their recommendations? Should you base rankings on the frequency that different proposals were mentioned? Should you give more weight to ideas coming from groups with more proximity and experience with the issue? How does the feasibility of each suggestion play into the decision about priority setting? How about their fit with existing services? How should the "felt needs" of the community be reconciled with the "hard data" of health status indicators? What about the trade-offs between feasibility and importance? What do you do with items that you know will antagonize the mayor, like a needle exchange program? Where is the formula for deciding? "In priority setting," Carl Taylor states, "judgment and wisdom are most needed, together with a unique ability to synthesize the numerous relevant details. It is the part of the planning process which is usually considered most intuitive."[25]

Finally, let us consider the specific area where theory is expected to offer the most help: producing more effective interventions. The community is concerned about violence, especially violence against women. The health promoter does her research and finds a few articles presenting evidence of the effectiveness of the Health Belief Model in violence prevention. But after reviewing the list of confirmed, theoretically derived behavioral risk factors, she comes to the uncomfortable conclusion that these constructs are terribly shallow. She is reminded of the words of Charles Anderson: "The general laws (which, to the positivists, it is their prime responsibility to produce) turn out too often to be curiously banal and trivial."[26] What does she say after telling her audience about their susceptibility and the severity of getting beaten? Where is the theory to guide her in giving women the courage to confront their abusers, the prudence to think about the best timing, or the wisdom to know when to leave? Where is the theory to help men see the need to bring their lives more closely in tune with visions of justice, integrity, shame, and self-control? What does theory tell her about confronting community apathy toward the inferior status of women? poverty? discrimination? Where is the theory to show her the ideal about how men and women should relate?

These examples seem to me to convey the reality of a health promoter's work-a-day world more accurately than the image of proficient experts operating with a set of highly specialized technical skills for implementing scientifically proven interventions. There is indeed a gap between theory and practice in health promotion today, but it arises because theory—based on the positivist model—has little to offer practitioners. Doing health promotion is *not* like doing medical procedures. It takes a different frame of mind, a different kind of understanding, a different process of making decisions. The goal of discovering the psychological equivalents of high blood pressure measures and developing an analogue of the physician's desk reference (PDR) to look up effective remedies with prescribed dosages is a false god, no matter how appealing the possession of such power might seem. Health promotion is not a set of technical scientific procedures. It is an ethical and political process of working together with fellow citizens in the struggle to come up with a clearer, more cogent, and more compelling conception of human well-being, an ideal toward which people want to work together to realize.

So, the health promoter decides to speak up in the meeting, confront the mayor, stick to the predetermined curriculum for the workshop but follow up on the student's question, maintain her professional distance rather than answer questions about her personal struggles with alcohol and unsafe sex, but pass on the scientific journals and instead convene a group of community residents to talk about what they think can be done about violence against women. How do we know whether she made the correct (true? best? most effective? most ethical?) decision? What are the warrants of practical reason?

THE WARRANTS OF PRACTICAL REASON

To cut to the conclusion, the warrants for claiming that a practical proposition is valid, that some decision is the right course of action, lie in securing the agreement and assent of others. Hoy and McCarthy elaborate, making a subtle but important point: it is not *because* we agree that we can claim that some statement about practical matters is true, but rather, we reach agreement because we have reasonable grounds for granting its validity.[27]

So, what are we talking about here? The kinds of questions addressed by practical reason are questions of the following order. What is a good way of life for people? What are important values to live by? Is it better for teenagers to remain sexually abstinent, or to be sexually active while protected by contraceptive devices? Is it better for people to have never experienced any mind-altering drug (including alcohol), only certain mind-altering drugs, or to practice moderation in their use? How much time should people devote to exercise and how much time should they give to their families, children, or community? Are societies that tolerate high levels of poverty and inequality the kind of societies we want to live in and be members of? What is the correct answer? How do we *know* that whatever we decide is *true*?

For Taylor and others, questions about the validity of value judgments stem from a categorical mistake. We have confused "the question of what something *is*" with "the question of how it is *known*."[28] We struggle to say something meaningful about the good life for human beings, to present a richer, more fully articulated vision of how we can share this space on earth more decently, but we are immediately greeted by the modern skeptical mind, "How do you know that what you claim is true?" Well, we don't, at least not with the same degree of certainty that we know the force of gravity or the reactions of chemicals in test tubes. But that does not mean that such attempts are irrational, arbitrary, groundless, personal opinions. Nor does it mean that we should give up the attempt to say what those values are in the most fully developed exposition we can muster simply because we do not have independent, objective criteria to say with absolute certainty that we know this description—this effort, this account, this time—is true and unmistaken. To those who persist in challenging the claims of practical reason, Taylor responds, "Now one, and perhaps the only, sane response to this would be to say that such uncertainty is an ineradicable part of our epistemological predicament."[29]

As noted earlier, the main legacy of positivism is an enduring belief in the dichotomy between objective facts and subjective opinion.[30] In rebuttal, Appleby and others suggest that there is a third option, something in between scientific proof and idle speculation.[31] Anderson provides a good illustration of this reasoning process:

> Like most of the elemental notions—justice, integrity—that guide our moral life, we do not have a sharply discriminating, operational definition ready at hand. Rather, we proceed by mutually intelligible intimations, affirming this, denying that, each claim suggesting an aspect of the whole that we vaguely discern but cannot readily grasp. . . . This is what makes reasoned argument possible. We persist in trying to persuade our antagonists that there is some crucial element of the matter at hand that their case neglects, and we proceed in the good faith that if we show them this perceptively, if we *illuminate* them, they may change their minds. And for our part, we presume that we may *learn* from the deliberation, which is to say, we keep open, and positively, the prospect that the case we are now earnestly making we will come to recognize as inadequate, because we will see a more significant, a larger truth in the matter.[32]

In thinking about the good life for human beings, the point of reasoning is to gain clarity, not to claim certainty.

The practice of putting forward, considering, and accepting arguments for or against a proposal is the core of practical reason.[33] In dialogue, one tries to get people to change their position by pointing out the contradictions, confusions, and points neglected in their position,[34] while at the same time remaining open to the possibility that one's own stance may need to be reexamined in light of the reasoning put forward in exchange. People are motivated to make claims and to press their case because they are convinced that their position can be supported by convincing reasons.[35] In seeing things in a new light, confusion is dissipated, the pieces fall into place, and our ideas gain coherence.

In the realm of *praxis*, there are no formal procedures comparable to the double-blind, randomized control trial. The warrants for claims are those used by judges and historians. A judge weighs her knowledge of law, the case history of precedents, her interpretation of the moral principles enshrined in the law, her insights regarding other relevant principles that should be brought to bear, and her understanding of the particulars in the case before her. She lays out her reasoning process, the relevant evidence and justifications that support her decision. They do not "prove" the decision is right, but we recognize that it is not arbitrary and capricious either. Similarly, the historian describes a pattern of events, presents evidence supporting an interpretation, and makes a case regarding the causes of a momentous decision, say, the invasion of Poland. His judgment is supported by reasons which the reader will consider more or less compelling. This never amounts to a proof, but it is still quite rational.

So, if there are no a priori, scientific criteria for proving that some practical statement is true (i.e., the wisdom of pursuing one course of action over another), how are we supposed to come to any conclusions about what we should do? Bernstein answers, "There is no test for the adequacy of an opinion, no authority for judging it, *other than the force of better public argument*."[36] Or, as Supreme Court Justice Oliver Wendall Holmes has written, "The best test of truth is the power of the thought to get itself accepted in the competition of the market."[37]

In the end, truth claims in matters of practical reason are redeemed through gaining the assent of others. The validity of judgment is established by eliciting the agreement and consensus of others. The warrants of practical reason are thus finally rooted in dialogue. Hannah Arendt expresses the point: "The power of judgment rests on potential agreement with others, and the thinking process which is active in judging something is not, like the thought process of pure reasoning, a dialogue between me and myself, but finds itself always and primarily, even if I am quite alone in making up my mind, in anticipated communication with others with whom I know I must finally come to some agreement."[38] Claims about the good life are true to the extent that others agree that it is a kind of life they want to work to bring about. Should people exercise more? The claim is true to the extent that people agree, to the extent that they become convinced that it is something worthwhile toward which they want to devote their time and energies. To the extent that people think that it interferes with other pursuits they consider more important, then health promoters need to listen and think about whether they have given us good reason to agree. Along these lines, in the exercise of practical reason, let us turn now to reevaluating the goals of health promotion, the topic of the next chapter.

6

HEALTH AND WELL-BEING

> "They have their little pleasure for the day and their little plea-
> sure for the night: but they respect health. 'We have discov-
> ered happiness,' say the Ultimate Men and blink."
> —Fredrich Nietzsche, *Thus Spoke Zarathrustra*

There is something sick about how we think about health. "When polled, Americans commonly list health at the top of their preoccupations, ahead of love, work,
or money, and identify good health ahead of any other alternative, including love,
as the chief source of happiness," writes Michael Ignatieff in his essay "Modern
Dying." "The gyms, squash courts, Nautilus rooms, swimming lanes, and saunas
of the big cities resound with the thud and the grunt of the last men and women in
pursuit of their grail."[1] Health is now an integral part of popular concerns, with
plenty of bedside reading. Perusal of the health section of any bookstore reveals
innumerable books on diet, exercise, stress, recovery, vitamins, biofeedback, and
on and on. Indeed, health books have replaced philosophy books as guides to the
good life. True to Nietzsche's portents, we seem to have reduced the idea of the
human good to the glow of physical fitness and the ideals of self-knowledge and
self-control to a dawn-to-dusk regimen of diet and exercise. We have a bad case
of hypochondria.

The source of such abundance [of health concerns] may lie finally in our cultural
fixation on health. People in every era, of course, have sought remedies for what ails
them, from Roman baths to Chinese herbs. Yet never before have average citizens
been at the mercy of electronic media desperate to fill airtime with the latest medical
information; never have people faced the daily deluge of health-related advertising
subsidized by hospitals, insurance carriers, and huge international pharmaceutical

companies. Every major newspaper hires a health reporter. Each new issue of *Nature*, *Science*, and the *New England Journal of Medicine* gets prereleased to TV networks that scan it for breathtaking stories on health, no matter how small the study or how preliminary the data. It is tempting, if ultimately erroneous, to identify the distinctive postmodern illness as a culture-wide hypochondria that takes the form of health worship.[2]

Despite burgeoning investments, surveys reveal a declining satisfaction with personal health across the country.[3] What is going on?

Health, like justice, power, integrity, and any other elemental notions of human concern, is a deeply ambiguous concept. We do not have a single sharply discriminating operational definition ready at hand. "Nevertheless," the ethicist Daniel Callahan remarks, "how a society thinks about those old questions, the way it frames the issues, the means by which it acts on rough-hewn answers can, and usually does, make all the difference in the lives of people."[4]

This chapter addresses the ends of health promotion. It takes initial steps toward articulating a deeper understanding of human well-being. If a characteristic failing of instrumental reason is the tendency to abdicate responsibility for reflecting on ends and to restrict itself to means, and if practical reason is the antidote, then it is time to begin thinking more about the kinds of lives and kinds of societies that constitute the good life for human beings.

As a starting point for this discussion, well-being will be defined in terms of integrity, of living one's life in accordance with values that matter. It is a life of becoming, not a discrete fixed outcome. It is striving to see more clearly the values that define the kind of person one wants to be and the kind of society we want to live in together. It is seeking to bring individual and collective actions more closely in line with those values, and thus, becoming more well integrated. Please note: because practical reasoning recognizes that values may well conflict with one another and that different people may come to different conclusions about the values that give their lives meaning, purpose, and happiness,[5] there is no single prescription, no one single definition of the good life pronounced here, other than a life of integrity, of living a life worth living. That is to say, the kinds of lives that constitute the good life for human beings are plural in number.[6]

As we shall see in the final chapter, certain social conditions are prerequisite to attaining individual well-being. Because material conditions are often harsh, haphazard, and plagued with adversities that no amount of individual effort could possibly overcome, the prospects for individual well-being are dependent on the justice of social conditions to an extent that we rarely consciously appreciate. While sometimes losing sight of it, we continue to uphold an ideal of justice that beckons us to arrange our social institutions such that people are not subjected to undeserved hardships or deprivations. Community well-being is here defined in terms of justice—the good order of institutions that insures that lives of integrity are the surest route to human fulfillment.

This chapter lays out a framework for rethinking the sources of human well-being based on the concept of a virtue. This framework will be used to reconceptualize the work of health promotion, one characterized by a recognition of the inextricable relationship between means and ends. Rather than viewing health as something that can be produced through the application of effective techniques, well-being may be better thought of as a way of being in the world, a kind of presence in which participation in certain kinds of social practices promotes—and other practices retard—the realization of human flourishing. This framework holds that well-being is realized through engaging in social practices that cultivate the virtue (or disposition) of mindfulness, self-knowledge and self-possession.

THE MYTHS OF HYGEIA AND ASCLEPIUS

According to the biologist René Dubos, there are two competing conceptions of health that have ancient roots.[7] These different understandings evolved in classical Greece in the divine cults of Hygeia and Asclepius. Hygeia was the goddess of well-being and "symbolized the belief that men could remain well if they lived according to reason. . . . She continued to symbolize the virtues of a sane life in a pleasant environment, the ideal of *mens sana in corpore sano*."[8] Hygeia stood for " 'living well,' or more precisely, a 'well way of living.' "[9] In this classical understanding, health was defined in terms of virtues and thus understood to be both a cause and an effect of itself. Leon Kass explains, "The Greek terms suggest that health is connected with the way we live and perhaps imply that health has largely an inner cause. Indeed, it seems reasonable to think of health understood as 'living well' or 'well-habited' as the cause of itself. Just as courage is the cause of courageous action, and hence also of courage—for we become brave by acting bravely—so 'living well' *is* health, is the *cause* of health, and is *caused by* health."[10] But from the fifth century on, devotion to Hygeia gradually gave way to that of the healing god, Asclepius.

Asclepius was the first physician in Greek legend. He "achieved fame not by teaching wisdom but by mastering the use of the knife and the knowledge of curative virtues of plants." His cult grew in stature because, Dubos writes, "to ward off disease or recover health, men as a rule find it easier to depend on healers than to attempt the more difficult task of living wisely."[11] Down through the ages, the myths of Hygeia and Asclepius have set the terms through which we have thought about health: "The myths of Hygeia and Asclepius symbolize the never ending oscillation between two different points of view in medicine. For worshipers of Hygeia, health is the natural order of things, a positive attribute to which men are entitled if they govern their lives wisely. . . . More skeptical, the followers of Asclepius believe that the chief role of the physician is to treat disease, to restore health by correcting any imperfections caused by accidents of birth or of life."[12]

Since the World Health Organization (WHO)'s declaration in 1948 that health is "a state of complete physical, mental, and social well-being and not merely the absence of disease," public health professionals have generally accepted the equation of health and well-being. Yet at the heart of the WHO definition beats an age-old ambiguity. In its modern form, "the basic dilemma seems to be whether health is a concept that can be defined objectively and technically, or whether it is a concept that refers finally and decisively to a quality of human experience that cannot be reduced to physiological processes."[13] Put another way, is "health" a descriptive term, or is it a normative concept?[14] Are we "well" when we measure up to a set of clearly defined indicators? Or does the concept refer to an evolving understanding of the values and ideals now packed into the term "social well-being?" Or, perhaps more to the point, what is the connection between these two understandings of health and well-being? How can we, as a society, have what appears to be a fairly passionate regard for physical fitness, evident in the profusion of workout videos, joggers, and smoking bans, while at the same time, have among the highest rates in the world of drug abuse, teen pregnancy, obesity, poverty, violence, homelessness, and infant mortality? What does this tell us about our level of wellness?

These indicators are outward manifestations of disturbances in well-being, two opposing reactions to an underlying malaise: on the one hand, the adulation of physical fitness, seeking happiness in a regimen of diet and exercise,[15] and on the other, a despairing view of the seeming meaninglessness of it all that mocks idolization of living longer through reducing heart disease. Plato once said that it is impossible to heal the body without at the same time treating the soul. Modern scientific medicine has conquered most infectious diseases and many types of biological breakdowns, but it is ill-equipped for the task of diagnosing and treating ailments of the soul, problems that stem from our desires and the choices we make about how we want to live our lives.[16]

As Weber intently perceived, it is a paradox of the modern era that, as technical capacities for treating the body have become more powerful, sociocultural capacities for discerning values that matter and ways of life worth living have deteriorated. Modern ailments are marked, Nussbaum observes, by "diseases of thought, judgment, and desire. . . . For society is not in order as it is; and, as the source of most beliefs and even of their emotional repertory, it has infected them with its sicknesses. The upbringing of youth is held to be deformed in various ways by false views about what matters: by excessive emphasis, for example, on money, competition, and status."[17] With the shift in the nature of contemporary ailments, we may recall the forgotten counsel, "Medicine heals the sicknesses of the body, but wisdom rids the soul of its sufferings."[18] The task for health promotion today is to take on the challenge of salvaging values, judgment, and reasoned reflection on the quality of our desires.

THE DIFFERENCE AND RELATIONSHIP
BETWEEN HEALTH AND WELL-BEING

To open a discussion about the ends of health promotion, I want to recall a classical distinction between health and well-being. These two concepts have become conflated in modern use, as in the World Health Organization (WHO) definition, and as a consequence, we find ourselves stuck with a terribly impoverished notion of human well-being, one reduced to health status indicators such as morbidity and mortality rates. If many people are not sure that life has anything more meaningful to offer, then devoting their lives to regimens of physical fitness may seem as worthwhile as any other pursuit. Others will find it difficult to make progress in reducing problems like drug abuse, violence, STDs, etc., unless they can reconnect with values that make life more meaningful, reasons that make life worth living and living well. To confront the challenges now facing the field, we need to rethink the terms and conditions of human well-being. There is no better starting point than Aristotle.

Aristotle made a consistent distinction between "health" and "well-being." Health (*holos*) referred to biological functioning, but "well-being" was denoted by the Greek term, *eudamonia*, which may also be translated as "flourishing," "happiness," "blessedness," or "prosperity." In Aristotle's writings, well-being is the ultimate good, the *telos* [end, goal] of all human activity guided by reason. As such, it is categorically distinct from "natural goods" or "goods *simpliciter*," such as health and wealth.[19] Health, for example, is too dependent on fate, fortune or luck; it was unthinkable to Aristotle to leave the prospects of living a good life to chance, outside of human powers to effect. So, in Aristotle's view, health and wealth were mere instrumental goods. They are sought not for their own sake, but only because they supply a means to bring about some other desired state. Viewing them as instrumental goods, Aristotle thought that their pursuit could in fact sometimes be harmful, materially and morally, as when individuals place a higher priority on pursuing wealth or health than on living an honorable life.[20] Well-being, however, is what he saw as the highest goal of human activity, that which is sought for its own sake, that toward which all intentional, purposive, reasoned actions are ultimately directed.[21] It is, by definition, complete in itself, not sought for the sake of attaining some other end.

In Aristotle's schema, the *telos* of rational human activity is to bring about well-being, happiness, the good life for human beings. What is the good life? Aristotle characterized human flourishing as a life of excelling in those functionings that are distinctively human.[22] In his words, "How should a human being live? In accordance with all the forms of good functioning that make up a good human life."[23] What does this mean? By way of analogy, we call a knife a *good* knife if it cuts well, because the function of a knife is to cut. So too, we would call a human life a good life if it did that which is its defining function—what we do that makes us who we are—most excellently.

At this point, Aristotle's framework per se encounters insurmountable difficulties; his metaphysic on the cosmological order is no longer plausible in light of modern understandings. To update the framework and complete the analogy, Taylor offers a more defensible candidate: "What is distinctively human is the power to *evaluate* our desires, to regard some as desirable and others as undesirable."[24] Taylor's position is not dependent on any transcendental metaphysical claims about the essence of human nature. Rather, it is an understanding grounded in history and in the exchange of reasons and arguments among human beings. It is open to challenge and revision, not absolute and final, but none the worse for that. It provides a provisional—yet more than adequate—foundation for opening discussions about the good life for human beings.

In Taylor's account, "It seems to be peculiarly characteristic of humans, however, that they are able to form . . . second-order desires. . . . Our desires are classified in such categories as higher and lower, virtuous and vicious, more or less fulfilling, more or less refined, profound and superficial, noble and base."[25] The goal of health promotion is to improve health, but the underlying source of most major contemporary threats to health lie in disturbances in human judgment. Therefore, to promote health, the task before the field is to promote practices that enable people to excel in evaluating their desires. The good life is the life spent seeking clearer understandings of values we think important to realize and striving to live our lives more closely attuned to those values. The end of health promotion is, accordingly, the life of integrity. "Integrity properly denotes *both wholeness and soundness*," Selznick writes. "To have integrity is to be unmarred by distortion, deception, or other forms of disharmony and inauthenticity."[26] In a moment, we will see that cultivating certain virtues (or dispositions) is essential for achieving integrity, both causing and constituting living more closely in tune with values that matter.

This framework offers a thought-provoking alternative to the health status indicator model that now dominates thinking in health promotion. The distinction between health and well-being may also help sort out several issues that frequently get confused when these terms are collapsed or equated. For example, the distinction helps us to see how health enthusiasts may have confused a state of physical fitness with the ideal of well-being. In the absence of any higher goals, Nietzsche's "Ultimate Men" think they have discovered happiness. But, as Aristotle observed, a preoccupation with physical fitness can become as harmful, materially and morally, as its neglect. The distinction helps us to be clearer about how it is that we can consider specimens of perfect physical health as sick, unwholesome, and maladjusted. Most of us still think the life of Martin Luther King, Jr. more worth emulating, for example, than the life of Dennis Rodman, however much "healthier" Rodman might be.

Conversely, we can think of many examples of people who might suffer a disease but whom we still regard as living well: "A woman who has multiple sclerosis who has come to terms with her condition and is leading a full and productive life within certain limitations. A man dying of bowel cancer who peacefully approaches his own death with the support of his family might be said to have a very healthy approach despite the fact that his life is coming to an end."[27]

The distinction may also help us to understand why the general public may not, at times, be as enamored with the field's entreaties regarding diet, exercise, and nonsmoking as official plans would have them. If health qua biological fitness is indeed better understood as merely an instrumental good—that which is sought only for the sake of attaining some higher goal—then it becomes easier to see why some people may not understand the value of getting fit until they have a stronger sense of what they are getting fit for. Why live longer unless there is something worth living for? Why should I give up my little pleasures now?

Finally, reviving the distinction between health and well-being challenges the way we think of the work of health promotion. Rather than viewing our work as a set of technical procedures designed to eliminate risk factors, a shift in thinking would entail seeing well-being as a process of becoming, in which the ends are not independent of the means. Well-being is realized through living well, through engaging in social practices that embody the values we wish to bring into being.

MINDFULNESS: THE VIRTUE OF WELL-BEING

The concept of a virtue—once we get past a slightly archaic ring and prudish connotations—offers an innovative framework for reconceptualizing the work of health promotion. Here, well-being is not an outcome that can be produced through reducing risk factors. It is, instead, viewed as an integral way of life. Well-being is living a life of integrity. It is the process of actualizing an integrated mode of perceiving and acting.

There are four interlocking parts in this framework for health promotion: virtues, social practices, internal goods, and institutions. I will start by defining each of these four parts, beginning with two definitions of virtues.

The first is from the philosopher Bernard Williams. A virtue is "a disposition of character to choose or reject actions because they are of a certain ethically relevant kind"[28] where "character" refers to the relatively persistent forms that a person's motivation takes.[29] As such, Pincoffs notes that virtues "are not just tendencies to act in certain ways, but also to feel, to think, and to react."[30] Kosman elaborates, "virtues are cultivated and not chosen in any simple sense, for it is not as a direct result of calculation, deliberation, or resolution, or any other relatively simple mode of human activity that we become courageous, temperate, or wise. We become these through a process of *ethismos*, or habituation, through the habitual acting out and embodying of those actualizations which the dispositions are dispositions towards."[31] As a result of cultivating certain virtues, over time, with habit and practice, our feelings typically change, becoming more responsive, more in harmony with what we wish to become.[32]

The philosopher Alasdair MacIntyre provides a more exacting and demanding definition:

> A virtue is an acquired human quality the possession and exercise of which tends to enable us to achieve those goods which are internal to practices and the lack of which effectively prevents us from achieving any such goods. . . . By a "practice" I am going to mean any coherent and complex form of socially established cooperative human activity through which goods internal to that form of activity are realized in the course of trying to achieve those standards of excellence which are appropriate to, and partially definitive of, that form of activity, with the result that human powers to achieve excellence, and human conceptions of the ends and goods involved, are systematically extended.[33]

MacIntyre's point about goods internal to social practices brings us back to the relationship between means and ends. MacIntyre offers the example of chess playing to illustrate the difference between internal and external goods. The internal good of chess playing is improving the level of play, through cultivating one's analytic skills, strategic imagination, competitive intensity, and the like. External goods, however, consist of things such as money, fame, or status, the accumulation of which in themselves does not make one a better player. The distinction calls attention to the fact that the pursuit of external goods is not directly linked to the development of human capacities. It is easy to think of situations where the means become corrupted, for instance, cheating to win a chess game. External rewards can be acquired without developing and extending human capacities. In contrast, when seeking to realize the internal goods of a social practice, cheating would defeat the purpose of participation. Just so, losing weight through diet pills does not enable us to realize the internal goods of self-knowledge, self-discipline, dignity, and integrity.

Now we can put the pieces together. Virtues are dispositions, relatively persistent tendencies to feel, to think, and to act in certain ways directed toward realizing well-being. Virtues imbue one's outlook on life with consistent, characteristic ways of perceiving and acting on felt desires. Virtues are cultivated through habitually participating in certain types of social practices. Social practices must be organized around internal goods in order to foster the development of virtues. In the last step, institutions are the conservators of internal goods. They preserve our understanding of the value of internal goods; they protect us from corrupting social practices, as when they are reorganized around external rewards. So, finally, it takes good institutions to make good people.[34] In this framework, the sources of individual and community well-being lie in institutional practices that cultivate certain virtues tied to the realization of internal goods. With a sketch of the major elements now in place, we can take a closer look at those virtues most relevant to health and well-being.

For Aristotle, well-being was realized through living a life expressed in four primary virtues—justice, courage, prudence, and *sophrosyne*. The virtues most relevant to health promotion are the virtues of *sophrosyne* and *civitas*. (*Civitas* is discussed in the next chapter.) The most common English translation of *sophrosyne* is "temperance," although etymologically, it comes from the Greek meaning, "saving *phronesis*" or "soundness of mind." Drew Hyland offers a delightful example of how we might go about defining the concept.

The Virtue of Philosophy is Hyland's exposition of Plato's *Charmides*, a classic Socratic dialogue on the virtue of *sophrosyne*.[35] The dialogue opens with Socrates encountering the youthful Charmides and asking him how he can account for his "wisdom or beauty or both." He answers that people become wise and beautiful through exhibiting the virtue of *sophrosyne* and the rest of the dialogue is taken up with trying to define what this means. What is it that a *sophron* person does that makes them *sophrosyne*?

Charmides's first answer is that to be *sophron* means to be quiet and calm. Socrates replies that this cannot be so, for what kind of life would that be. If we were always cool, calm, and collected and never without some passion, life would be dull and boring, and hence not worth living. Charmides's second and third responses fare no better. His second answer is that it means modesty, and his third, minding one's own business. Socrates punctures these trial balloons in short order, but then the dialogue moves onto a more abstract plane. Eventually, after several rather intricate arguments, the discussants come to the position that to be *sophron* means to have self-knowledge. To attain wisdom or beauty or both, one must be "aware of what one knows and does not know."

But, the dialogue continues, self-knowledge is not the same as knowledge about things or facts. Self-knowledge entails not only understanding the way things are, but it can only come about through seeking to grasp ideals about the ways things ought to be too. Who we are is not something that is fixed and frozen, but rather we are always in a process of becoming. To attain self-knowledge thus requires remaining open, questioning the way things are, reexamining who we are in light of who we want to be. In Socrates's most famous words, "The unexamined life is not worth living." Thus, the dialogue concludes, *sophrosyne* is finally a disposition of "interrogative wonder." It is, Hyland concludes, best defined and translated as "responsive openness."

Nussbaum's account is equally refreshing. In Aristotle's work, the virtue of *sophrosyne* is essential for the harmonious management of bodily appetites. Aristotle saw two potent tendencies in human beings: an "innate appetite for pleasures" and an "acquired belief about the good." The first pertains to *orexis* (desire) and the second, *logos*, relates to rational reasoning. Nussbaum then explains, "The state of a person in which belief about the good is in control is called *sophrosone*. The state in which the appetite that draws us toward pleasure is in control is called simply *hubris* or wantonness."[36] A person lacking *sophrosyne* mindlessly pursues pleasures. In contrast, the *sophron* person is fully aware of his appetites: he will enjoy food, drink, and sex in appropriate measure, but not in excess. Thus, this virtue is the disposition to be sensitive to the stirrings of desire within us and to put them in proper perspective. To be temperate is to find the right balance, so that one does not characteristically long for the wrong food, drink, or other sensual gratifications at the wrong time in the wrong amount. *Sophrosyne* is here defined as rational self-possession and characterized as the harmonious relationship of intense passion under perfect control. It is contrasted with *mania*, which involves the loss of insight, the tendency toward excess, and an unreflective, regardless lack of control.

Bellah brings the discussion into contemporary terms. In a powerful essay on caring in contemporary America, he calls for the replenishment of "mindfulness" and "paying attention." Bellah asserts that problems arise when our attention gets disturbed. On the one hand, "attention is how we use our psychic energy, and how we use our psychic energy determines the kind of self we are cultivating, the kind of person we are learning to be. When we are giving our full attention to something, when we are really attending, we are calling on all our resources of intelligence, feeling, and moral sensitivity."[37] When we devote full attention to our life projects, we extend the potentialities of our selves and our relationships. In so doing, we reaffirm ourselves in the larger contexts that give meaning to our lives. Paying attention also means that we do not close our eyes to the world around us and its ills.

Yet all of us suffer, to one degree or another, from attention disorders. Bellah continues, "When we are doing something we 'have to do,' but our minds and our feelings are somewhere else, our attention is alienated. In such situations of disordered or alienated attention our self-consciousness is apt to be high. We may suffer from anxiety, or today's common complaint, 'stress'. . . . We attend but fitfully—inattentively, so to speak—and therefore we are not cultivating ourselves or our relationships with others. Rather we may be building up strong desires to seek distractions when we have free time."[38] We seek out distractions—alcohol, drugs, restless channel flipping, promiscuous sex, working out, etc.—to ward off the anxiety and stress that come from participating in activities in a distracted, distraught manner, present in body but not in spirit. Bellah concludes, "Our argument is that if we are going to be the kind of persons we want to be and live the kinds of lives we want to live, then attention and not distraction is essential."[39]

Sophrosyne is mindfulness about bodily appetites and other first-order desires.[40] It is a disposition to pay attention, to become more aware, more self-conscious about them, and to put them in perspective, to see them in the context of the kind of person one wants to become. It is both the means and the end of human well-being. We become well by becoming more mindful, and we cannot experience well-being without being mindful, without self-knowledge. It is both a cause and a constituent element of a life of integrity. It is a clear conscience, contentment, self-acceptance over having lived life well. On the other side of this same coin, the absence of this disposition is the condition of being obtuse, lacking insight, being insensitive, inattentive, out of sync. It is the loss of control, the loss of self-possession, where actions are driven by compulsive urges. It is being bothered by something we can't quite put our finger on and responding inappropriately. It is acting irresponsibly, in the literal sense of not having the ability to respond well to felt desires.

For example, I often misinterpret being exhausted from work as the need for food, when what I really need is to rest and to reevaluate whether I want to be the kind of person who gets caught up in the rat race of getting ahead. When we are inattentive or unmindful, we might be angry about something that happened at work, but we take it out on our spouse. Or we suppress something that is bothering us about how we are getting along with our partner, but wind up yelling at our children. We are upset about the way someone is treating us, but we eat too much in the misguided attempt to feel better, more satisfied. We are pressured to cut corners at work, but, burying the emotion, we feel like having a drink. We delude ourselves. We lust after a colleague, feeling the urge to make a pass, forgetting we are married with children. We make love and, in the heat of the moment, we forget that having a child at this time would not be good for anyone involved. We get angry and say something stupid, thoughtless, to a friend. We help ourselves to another serving or another glass of wine without thinking, compulsively mistaking the dulling of sensation for feelings of fulfillment. We foolishly think that plumping down in a chair in front of the television will restore the lost psychic energy from being pulled in too many directions at once, not attending to any of them well. We fill up our lives with distractions, neglecting to pay attention to whether we are becoming the kind of person we want to become.

Conversely, becoming more mindful is gaining self-knowledge. It is becoming more attentive, more aware of the full extent of the reasons for our acts, for the choices we make. It is not letting ourselves fall into self-deceit, ignoring or denying that we might be acting out of spite, gluttony, or greed. It is allowing the full range of our motivations to enter into our consciousness so we can better see if that is the kind of person we want to be, and deciding on another course of action if acting out of ill will is not how we like to think of ourselves. It is saving *phronesis*, making conscious choices, becoming more fully aware of what we are doing.

For health promotion, cultivating mindfulness would mean helping youth sort out what the urge to smoke is really all about for them. It is helping people put their desires for sex and drugs into perspective. It is talking about what the impulse to have unprotected sex with multiple partners means, trying to help them understand themselves better. It is a process of aiding people in becoming more responsible, of developing their capacity to see and to respond to inner impulses and outer pressures, of recognizing and evaluating felt desires, and of owning one's response to them. It is the conscious practice of striving to become more autonomous, more responsible, more well integrated.

The field has a responsibility to make people aware of what is known about the causes of biological breakdowns and their prevention and treatment. But from there our main concern must be to support people in improving their own capacities for practical autonomy. If we can help people become more mindful about their choices (in a process through which we are as likely to learn as they are), become clearer about the value of a particular course of action, and become more perceptive about whether initial inclinations proceed from misbegotten or misdirected motives which they may later regret (e.g., taking drugs to "get even" with their parents), then we will have done a lot.

RETHINKING THE SOURCES OF HUMAN WELL-BEING

The dominant image informing health promotion today is that people are impacted by discrete risk factors that cause them—or make them more likely—to take up unhealthy behaviors. The approach described here suggests rethinking both the means and ends of achieving human well-being. This section opens with a description of one contemporary threat to health, alcohol abuse, but reconsiders it in terms of the framework described in these pages.

Alcohol abuse is a serious public health problem, second only to smoking in terms of the number of lives lost prematurely each year. As we saw in Chapter 2, official plans to combat this problem have targeted identified risk factors such as perceived severity (Health Belief Model) and perceived social norms (Theory of Reasoned Action) to effect reductions in consumption. But what if this is not the way people make choices, that is, caused by independent, antecedent social–psychological variables? What if choices are much more complexly intertwined with one's character and an outlook permeating the whole of one's perceptions, passions, and sense of possibilities? In this perspective, the same stimulus would have different meanings for different people, meanings and interpretations linked to their sense of identity, of who they are and what is important to them. In the following passage, Herbert Fingarette provides a rich illustration of how we might reconceptualize the ways people experience problems with alcohol in the terms outlined in this chapter. The account carries major implications for rethinking how we might restore their sense of well-being. The reader will note the correspondence between Fingarette's description of "central activities" and that of social practices as described above.

> To say heavy drinking is a *central activity* for someone is to say that it is an activity of the same order for that person as my vocation is for me. Our central activities tell something about what we do with a meaningful portion of our time. Yet far more is at stake than the appropriation of time. For a central activity affects the style and nature of all aspects of our lives and interacts with all our other central activities. . . . [I]n an important sense, though each of us initially makes choices that eventually determine our central activities, once an activity becomes central it influences, inspires, or even seems to demand certain other choices that further define who we are, how we act, where we go, and what we value.
>
> In an analogous way, as heavy drinking becomes a central activity in the drinker's life, it shapes his or her daily schedule, friendships, domestic life, and occupational choices. Heavy drinkers tend to organize their lives to minimize contact with people who frown on drinking or condemn excessive drinking. And they tend to seek out people and situations that evoke and stimulate drinking—choices reinforced by various socially acceptable settings, rituals, and justifications for drinking. . . .
>
> [M]ost of the time we are like the investor or the architecture buff, with our central activities continuously conditioning our perceptions of persons, places, and events. Our way of life is not simply something we bring to situations; over time, our way of life develops its own power and momentum in defining situations and our responses to them.
>
> So a heavy drinker arrives for an informal party at a friend's house. While other guests scan the room to seek out the host or to notice the decor or the food, the heavy drinker immediately searches for the bar and winces if it is poorly equipped. And as guests begin to circulate to see who else has arrived, the heavy drinker notices one crony who has on occasion joined him for a few rounds at the neighborhood bar, and an eagle-eyed friend of his brother's, one who's sure to report disapprovingly on how much drinking went on at this party.[41]

This is a much more complex portrait of life in which it makes little sense to speak of causal or independent risk factors. Drinking is an integral part of a way of life, affecting all aspects, from one's daily schedule, to invitations accepted or declined, to how one sizes up a social gathering. Just as drinking can become a way of life, conditioning our perceptions of situations and the choices that appear to be available to us, so well-being is the obverse: living well, well-habited, made possible by acquiring a disposition that imbues one's feelings, one's perceptions and motivations, shaping one's desires and choices of activities. In a different frame of mind, health promoters might think about the kinds of social practices that engender attentiveness, mindfulness, responsive openness. It is a different practice, yet one for which we have a few excellent examples at hand.

After millions and millions of dollars of research, it is remarkable that the best known treatment for alcohol abuse is Alcoholics Anonymous (AA).[42] Fingarette's description and the analysis outlined in these pages may help us to understand better why this is the case. The model of AA is a group of people who voluntarily come together to discuss issues of common concern, meeting in open public spaces, such as church basements and community centers. There are no scientists, no skilled professionals, no therapists leading the session. Meetings usually start with an invitation for someone to propose a topic for discussion, an issue or concern with which the individual is now grappling. Frequently, the issue is initially inchoate, only dimly perceived, a nagging bother that the person who proposed it is struggling to understand. But as the discussion moves around the room, people share their insights, how it feels to them, how they see it, how they cope. Through this sharing, people gain new insight into their own troubles. They begin to see themselves from uncharacteristic angles, with restored perspective.[43] The sharing is a healing process. Their desires—at one time overwhelming—become transformed, reintegrated into a broader pattern of meaning in life.

Another model of social practices that cultivate the disposition of mindfulness is the feminist conscious-raising group.[44] It is this type of practice, I believe, that holds the most promise for the future of health promotion. It is a collective cooperative human activity aimed at realizing the good for human beings through fostering self-knowledge, autonomy, integrity, respect, responsibility, solidarity, and social action to expand the sphere of justice in this world. Without describing their work in terms put forward here, the National Black Women's Health Project is now putting this model into practice.[45]

Another example is an on-going experiment with the creation of workers' occupational health committees in Italy.[46] There workers establish their own specific groups based on their perceptions of the different working conditions and environments to which different types of workers are subjected. They keep workbooks to record information on the work process, the work environment, and the products used in the process. That information is discussed and analyzed by the group of workers. Workers can request technical assistance from experts of their choice, but whatever information they provide is subject to a process of mutual validation. "Findings are discussed, accepted, or rejected depending on whether the assembled workers feel they conform with their own feelings or perceptions. . . . Once the problem and its causes are discussed and defined by the workers themselves, the work group decides on the strategy to solve the problem."[47] Hancock and Minkler describe several other projects that appear to exhibit characteristics like those advocated here.[48]

Two final examples of on-going work in Holyoke close this chapter. The work of El Centro de Educacion durante El Embarazo (CEDE, the Center for Education during Pregnancy) is guided by the able leadership of the director, Gladys

Lebron. CEDE was established in response to concerns for the high rate of infant mortality, the low rate of women receiving adequate prenatal care, and the abysmally low rates of immunizations in Holyoke. The primary work of CEDE goes on in *charlas* (Spanish for "chats"). Gladys, a long-time resident of the community, is well-known and highly respected in the neighborhood where she lives and works. Gladys meets with small groups of women and men in the evenings in their homes, and over food and drink, these small groups discuss their concerns about pregnancy and the life awaiting their children. There are no theories, no operational objectives, no formulas for treatment, only people caring for one another and trying to work out the best that they can do in their circumstances in Holyoke here and now.

Although well versed about medical issues during pregnancy, Gladys never prepares a set program plan with measurable learning objectives. Instead, she puts a premium on being sensitive and responsive to the concerns that community members bring. She knows from experience that what people were interested in last week might change this week. The women talk about how they are getting along, and, on one level, the discussions are very pragmatic—finding childcare, arranging transportation, discussing different obstetricians and midwives, home births versus hospital deliveries. But, on another level, the dialogue is about expressing fears, expressing hopes, exploring issues in their marriages, their jobs, their experiences with the educational system, struggles with alcohol and other drugs, what sets things off and what helps them to keep it together. While ostensibly a perinatal project, Gladys finds herself working on housing issues, organizing tenants, sharing information about AIDS, helping neighbors get drug dealers out of their building. More importantly, she is fostering a sense of trust, community, and hope for a better world. Participants listen to one another, they respect each other, they care for one another. They are engaged in a social practice, cultivating the habit of paying attention to what matters.

Yet CEDE is not a totally coherent social practice. Certainly a language of virtues, social practices, and internal goods would sound strange to Gladys (although the values of *respeto*, *dignidad*, and *familia* frequently enter the discussions). With funding from the Department of Public Health, Gladys is constantly under pressure to identify and demonstrate the achievement of targeted outcomes—increased compliance in attending prenatal appointments, fewer premature births, fewer low birthweight babies, lower infant mortality rates. She understands the value of these outcomes, yet views them as only one small part of a larger set of issues that women in her community face. Promoting healthier births is not an end in itself. Gladys knows that the problem of infant mortality cannot be resolved without attending to the kind of life and kinds of choices these women have available to them. CEDE evolved naturally, growing out of implicit understandings of the nature of community life and human relationships. Gladys and her staff struggle constantly against the press for instrumental rationalizations—people who demand to know the cost-effectiveness of their activities—and they find the resources for articulating other values and other justifications for their work as threadbare as the fabric of society.

More self-consciously, the Holyoke Community Health Planning Commission explicitly aims to improve the quality of community life by engaging residents in discussion and reflection on the conditions for individual and community well-being in Holyoke. The goal of the Commission is the good life for community members, but it is a goal that we see being attained through action and practice that is itself ethical and political. The means of treating one another with mutual respect, reinforcing individual dignity and autonomy, fostering a moral climate of justice and solidarity are the ends we seek to establish. Drawing on the models of CEDE and other programs, the Commission is trying to create as much public space as possible to engage as many people as possible to think about, plan, and carry out actions to improve the quality of shared community life. The 24–member Commission has representatives from every health and human service agency in Holyoke, the school department, police department, and city council; we deliberately chose representatives from the mid-management stratum of their respective organizations, people with some clout but still close enough to the clientele served by their agency. Commission members meet with community members almost anywhere people come together: in waiting rooms of the health center, in elder centers, in religious classes, at the Girl's Club, in after-incarceration parole groups, in parent–teacher groups, in meetings of CEDE, in drop-in centers, at the YMCA, in after-school groups, in child care places, and in word-of-mouth community forums. We ask residents their concerns and invite them to join various ad hoc task forces set up to address the issues they see as important. Thus far, the Commission has been overwhelmed by the depth of despair; creating a renewed sense of hope will not be an easy task. Clearly, the Commission would like to see the rates of infant mortality, substance abuse, AIDS, and violence fall, but we believe that will not happen until people feel reconnected to a world they want to call their own.

TAKING STOCK

With the major elements of an alternative framework for thinking about health promotion now in place, it may be helpful to take brief stock of where we are now in the discussion. The origins of many contemporary health problems—drug abuse, violence, teen pregnancy, suicide, smoking, alcohol abuse, child abuse, obesity, and so on—lie in cultural disturbances in the foundations of human choice: judgments about desires, or what Taylor calls "strong evaluation." Clarifying values and strengthening the human capacity for making sound judgments are not amenable to technical, scientific interventions. (Indeed, the allocation of immense resources directed toward developing the capacity to control people's behavior is symptomatic of the modern moral morass.) Recuperating understandings of values that matter is an ethical–political process. It was Nietzsche's insight that an absolute faith in meta-narratives about God no longer gripped the modern imagination and at last humanity was going to have to accept responsibility itself for defining the values by which we want to live together on this planet.

The process of clarifying and strengthening common understandings of human values is possible only through mutual discussion, debate, and deliberation among citizens. Community health educators can promote these deliberations and nurture these capacities through convening public discussions about issues of common concern in open public spaces. Practical reason is the human faculty of wise judgment, which is essential for discerning values that matter and for making strong second-order evaluations of felt desires. The virtue of mindfulness is a disposition to be open and to become more self-aware, which is both a cause and a constituent part of achieving integrity. It is cultivated through participation in social practices that have the internal goods of dignity, autonomy, and responsibility. Mindfulness is essential to enable people to live more closely attuned to values that matter. The recommendation here is that the field of health promotion should reorient its practices along the lines of engaging community members in discussions about the kinds of institutional practices that will help all of us to see more clearly values that matter and bring our actions more in harmony with those values.

7

CIVILITY, TRUST, AND COMMUNITY WELL-BEING

In shifting the discussion to the community level, this chapter makes arguments parallel to those in the preceding one about both the sources and the obstacles to achieving a greater measure of social well-being. Problems on the social level—poverty, inequality, homelessness, discrimination, and the associated pathologies of crime, drug abuse, and violence—are seen to stem in large part from the same underlying disturbances in judgment, the same deterioration in our ability to discern values that matter, which leads to problems in putting individual desires into perspective and determining the kinds of values that will enable us to live together decently, and indeed flourish. On the social level, there is a similar second stream of events contributing to the decline in our ability to define values that matter: the degeneration of social practices, specifically, the sharp decline of participation in social and civic groups.

The antidote is the promotion of social practices that engage the faculty of practical reason in civil society. Cultivating the virtue of civility is essential to the attainment of social or community well-being. Just as we cannot comprehend individual well-being without a high level of self-awareness, so we cannot conceive of community well-being without a high level of civility. Civility is becoming more fully conscious of the complete range of community members' needs and desires. It is seeing one's individual wants in the context of our lives as members of society, membership that defines, in part, who we are. The cultivation of this virtue enables us to recognize and put into perspective the fact that we are simultaneously autonomous individuals *and* community members. Civility is cultivated through participation in the social practices of civil society. One key indicator of social well-being is the level of trust among community members. Trust is built on the expectation that people will act with integrity.

Drawing on the work of the political philosopher Michael Sandel, this chapter opens with a reprise of his analysis of the sources of contemporary discontents. After reviewing a number of other additional factors, the chapter focuses on the social practices contributing to the sense of modern malaise, especially the decline in participation in civil society. In an analysis based on the work of the political scientist Robert Putnam, the discussion examines the impact of the precipitous withdrawal from civic interaction that has occurred over the last 30 years. With the decline of civil society, the bonds of community, the bounds of solidarity, and people's appreciation of the overlap between self-interests and the common good have shriveled. In combination, the erosion of the philosophical foundations for reasoning about the common good and the decline in social participation mutually feed and exacerbate one another, breeding a climate of cynical mistrust and the consequent withdrawal of public support from programs and policies aimed at improving the quality of life in common. Reversing these trends will require a revitalization of civil society.

The chapter moves on to the role of civil society in cultivating civility and in strengthening the faculty of practical reason. A discussion of trust as an indicator of community well-being and the integrity of social interactions follows. The chapter closes with examples of the institutional practices in health promotion that erode and those that promote the cultivation of civility and the generation of trust.

PUBLIC LIFE IN A PROCEDURAL DEMOCRACY

In *Democracy's Discontent*, Sandel identifies two issues that sum up the sources of American malaise: "One is the fear that, individually and collectively, we are losing control of the forces that govern our lives. The other is the sense that, from family to neighborhood to nation, the moral fabric of the community is unraveling around us. These two fears—for the loss of self-government and the erosion of community—together define the anxiety of the age."[1] Sandel argues that the reigning public political philosophy, which he calls a "procedural" democracy, is both responsible for the generation of these woes and ill-equipped to alleviate them. In its stead, he recommends the revitalization of an older understanding of politics, civic republicanism, to come to terms with the discontents of these times.

Sandel provides a concise summary of these two opposing political philosophies. Under the terms of the political philosophy by which we now live, the guiding principle of liberalism is that government should be neutral toward the moral and religious views of its citizens. Since people disagree about the best way to live, government should not affirm any particular vision of the good life, but should, instead, provide a framework of rights that protects persons as free and independent selves with conflicting values and ends. Since this political philosophy asserts the priority of fair procedures over substantive ends, Sandel terms this type of public life the "procedural republic."[2]

The major rival political philosophy is civic republicanism. Central to civic republican philosophy is the idea that liberty depends on sharing in self-government. The kind of public life envisioned here entails active deliberations among fellow citizens regarding the plight of the community. But, Sandel explains, to deliberate well about the common good requires more than a respect for rights: "It requires knowledge of public affairs and also a sense of belonging, a concern for the whole, a moral bond with the community whose fate is at stake. To share in self-rule therefore requires that citizens possess, or come to acquire, certain qualities of character, or civic virtues."[3] To illustrate their respective differences, he highlights two major issues in these rival philosophies: the relation of the right to the good, and the definition of liberty.[4]

In societies guided by a procedural outlook, concern for individual rights takes precedence over concern for the common good. In polities inspired by a philosophy of civic republicanism, promoting the common good assumes precedence over maximizing the right to pursue individual self-interests. Elsewhere, Sandel describes the difference between these two ethical and political outlooks as follows: "Where the morality of right corresponds to the bounds of the self and speaks to that which distinguishes us, the morality of good corresponds to the unity of persons and speaks to that which connects us."[5] That is to say, a concern for rights reflects a concern for protecting that which differentiates and separates us from each other; a concern for the good reflects an interest in promoting that which unites us, in expanding the sphere of what we share in common. As Sandel's analysis indicates, modern American life is marked by the priority of individual rights over the common good, a reversal of their classical relationship. Taylor calls these same distinctions "procedural" versus "substantive" conceptions of morality (also, an "ethics of rules" versus an "ethics of caring"[6]), and he concludes with respect to the priority of one over the other that "there is no simple one-sided resolution to this conflict."[7]

With regard to liberty and self-government, in the liberal concern for the protection of individual rights, personal desires or wants are regarded as incorrigible.[8] Politically, individuals cannot be called mistaken about what they want. Yearnings well up inside individuals for whatever reasons, but the quality of their desires is not debatable nor subject to questioning by others (except as they impinge on their liberty). Hence, a neutral state exists to protect the satisfaction of felt desires. Liberty is defined negatively, as freedom from the interference of others.

The aim of the liberal state is to remove as many obstacles as possible that might impede individuals from their pursuit of happiness, however conceived.

In the civic republican view, by contrast, liberty is the exercise of self-government, people ruling themselves, exercising positive control over their lives. Here, the fact that someone is doing what he wants, in the sense of satisfying his strongest desire, is not considered liberation. Taylor explains: "A man who is driven by spite to jeopardize his most important relationship, in spite of himself, as it were, or who is prevented by unreasoning fear from taking up the career he truly wants, is not truly made more free if one lifts the external obstacles to venting his spite or acting on his fear."[9] In this view, to be truly free is to gain control over one's urges. People are not free if they are driven by their passions, by fits of rage, jealousy, fear, or licentiousness. Acting on overwhelming desires to eat or drink is not considered freedom. Freedom in the positive sense is the freedom to become the kind of person one thinks admirable. Extrapolated to the larger community, liberty in the republican view is collective control over common life. Here, the aim of government is to create those conditions that enable people to work together to realize the kind of society they want to live in together.

In tracing the roots of democracy's discontent, Sandel sees our current situation as characterized by an increasingly lopsided resolve favoring the protection of individual rights and a corresponding decline in the institutional wherewithal for generating a counterbalancing disposition toward caring for the common good. In his diagnosis, the greatest threat to our well-being currently lies in the cynicism and anomie engendered by the abdication of responsibility to articulate and clarify values we share in common.

In sum, modern American malaise stems from a preoccupation with individual rights to the neglect of nurturing a sense of belonging, a concern for the whole, and a respect for the social bonds of community. Sandel's analysis indicates that the sense of unraveling, the erosion of community, and the loss of self-government felt in modern life may be traced to the corruption of our political practices, which have increasingly become sheer instrumental, strategic processes for advancing self-interests. On a philosophical level, as confidence in our ability to discern rationally defensible understandings of the common good has waned, we have been drawn increasingly toward the idea that we need procedural guarantees. In the face of modern skepticism, rather than grapple with questions about substantive values, we have come to accept a system of procedural protections of individual rights. In Sandel's view, the quality of community life will continue to deteriorate unless we can salvage stronger, clearer understandings of the common good. The nation's discontents can best be resolved through recovering a public political philosophy oriented toward establishing and expanding the sphere of the common good and reviving the associated social practices of civic republicanism.

Many factors have contributed to a sociocultural climate preoccupied with fortifying individual rights to pursue their own self-interests and marked by declining concern for the common good. Throughout this book, I have tried to indicate the ways in which an unstinting commitment to the power of science to solve social problems relegates questions about ends, values, and the common good to the realm of the irrational, locating them somewhere outside the bounds of valid determinations. When values are reduced to brute subjective preferences and considered unamenable to rational analysis and conclusions, the idea that we can achieve reasoned agreement about values that matter becomes increasingly implausible, receding ever farther from the grasp of the modern scientific mind. When the epistemological foundations for coming to sound, defensible conclusions about the good are called into question, a framework of rights secured with procedural protections seems the only option. Under these conditions, the quest for a science of health promotion both reflects and reinforces a climate in which striving for ever more effective power seems the best and perhaps the only means of securing one's desired ends. In terms of institutional practices, health promotion does not now focus on fostering public discussions about the common good, but on developing more effective means for eliminating smoking, heart disease, drug abuse, etc. As a consequence, however, seeking power to control people's behavior provokes defensive reactions of mistrust toward its practitioners, which further erode the bonds of community, a point taken up below.

Many other factors contribute to the diminution in hope that we can achieve broader, more substantive, shared understandings of the common good. Bellah and his colleagues have amply documented America's long and deeply cherished spirit of individualism and the corresponding preference for negative freedom, the tendency to favor freedom from communal obligations.[10] This individualistic bent deters concerns for the common good. Yet these authors point out that the American passion for liberty and the pursuit of individual happiness has traditionally been stabilized by the cultural mores that made such an impression on DeToqueville—the "habits of the heart" borne of participation in community associations that sustain commitment to enhancing the quality of shared public life.

On other items, in what many might consider a surprising turn, several eminent scholars of a liberal-progressive persuasion, including Arthur Schlesinger, Jean Bethke Elshtain, and Todd Gitlan[11] among others, have recently excoriated the rise of "identity politics"—politics given over to venerating differences by race, gender, sexual orientation, etc.—in the breakup of the Left and dissolution of a common dream of a better world. In the politics of the 1990s, furious energies have been expended in attacks on claims about common interests and in elevating the differences that divide people. African-Americans, women, gays, and other groups are held to have incommensurable values and any questionings are met with reflex charges of racism, sexism, homophobia, etc. Consequently, the defense of rights has displaced dialogue about the common good on the progressive political agenda over the past two decades, a position friendly critics are now calling into question.

Other progressives, such as Benjamin DeMott, attribute the desiccation of the idea of a common good to the cynical example set by the elite "leader-class."[12] After recapping a damning litany of charges—from corporate lies about nicotine to Iran–Contra, to police brutality, to proof that racism is rife among oil company executives—DeMott concludes:

> "Uncivil" refusal by ordinary citizens to labor unpaid in the cause of points-of-light good works reflects, in one of its dimensions, the daily exposure of ordinary citizens to powerful anti-mutuality instruction from above—oblique but persuasive lessons on how to pull your oar ceaselessly for the benefit of Number One; how not to fret about hungry children in the street; how to feel good when, in the age of homelessness, a corporate bright boy spends $45 million on his one-family dwelling; how to avoid being suckered into caringness. The 'new incivility' needs to be recognized, in short, for what it is: a flat-out, justified rejection of leader-class claims for respect, a demand that leader class types start looking hard at themselves.[13]

An attitude of jaded resignation and retreat into private life is now perhaps the most widespread political position of the populace in contemporary American society.[14]

The obstacles presented by dishonest leaders, strained race relations, unbridled individualism, and an unceasing faith in technology to solve any problems we may face have been around since the beginnings of the American republic. Yet the solipsistic pursuit of self-interests has historically been balanced by an expansiveness of spirit conceived in community associations. DeToqueville was most impressed by the willingness of the American people to give their time and energy to social groups dedicated to improving the quality of community life. This willingness to engage with others has been severely tested in recent years.

CIVILITY AND CIVIL SOCIETY

In a thought-provoking article that has generated considerable national discussion, Harvard political scientist Robert Putnam attributes the fraying of the social fabric to "Bowling Alone." Putnam's research shows a steady decline in the numbers and percentage of people participating in social groups—groups of any kind, from Elks Lodges, to political and fraternal organizations, to bridge clubs, hobby groups, and bowling leagues. After rejecting other potential explanations—such as the increase in the number of women in the workforce, job relocations, higher divorce rates, suburban sprawl—Putnam lays the decline in social participation at one formidable doorstep: TV. Dating from its introduction in the 1950s, the more people have turned to watching television, the less they have joined social groups. As a consequence, Putnam elaborates, "The social fabric is getting thinner, our connections among each other are becoming visibly thinner. We don't trust one another as much. And, of course, that is behind the deterioration of political dialogue, the deterioration of public debate."[15] He concludes, "In America, at least, there is reason to suspect that this democratic disarray may be linked to a broad and continuing erosion of civic engagement that began a quarter-century ago. . . . High on America's agenda should be the question of how to reverse these adverse trends in social connectedness, thus restoring civic engagement and civic trust."[16]

Following the analyses by Sandel and Putnam, if we are concerned that the quality of community life is deteriorating and that contemporary public health problems are symptoms of this disintegration, then a vital part of the healing process will be nourishing the bonds of community and strengthening our mutual capacity to discern values that define the common good. In recent years, there has been a resurgence of interest in the role of civil society in response to these twin concerns.

Like many of the ideas encountered up to this point, the concept of civil society has a rich history. Taylor has traced the major milestones in its evolution.[17] In Aristotle's writings, civil society was synonymous with the *polis*, or political society, and was closely associated with the development of the virtues of prudence and self-rule. The concept took on new connotations starting in the early Middle Ages, as societal organization grew more complex and differentiated. When the church split off as an independent social entity, political society slowly came to be seen as but one form of social organization among others. With the rise of the quasi-independent feudal estates and later a market economy of guild and craft merchants, civil society increasingly came to be identified with those groups and organizations that were independent of state power and control.

The concept of civil society took on increasing significance in the eighteenth century with the elaboration of the idea of an autonomous "public" with its own "opinion," outside of official state political assemblies. In this emerging understanding, public opinion came to be recognized as genuinely "public" because it was formed through collective debate and discussion, and put forward as something people held in common. Interest in civil society has been spurred today most notably through the writings of Vaclav Havel, dramatist-philosopher-president of Czechoslovakia, who, among other things, attributes the fall of communism to the growth and flourishing of civil society.[18]

With this background, Taylor defines civil society as "that web of autonomous associations, independent of the state, which bind citizens together in matters of common concern, and by their mere existence or action, could have an effect on public policy."[19] These associations began in church groups, trade guilds, salons, and coffeehouses. They are now typically thought to include unions, churches, political movements, cooperatives, neighborhood associations, interest groups, and "societies for promoting this and that."[20] Civil society is made up of all those associations where people choose to come together to talk about issues of common concern.

This type of interaction—the social practice of direct face-to-face public meetings—is vital for cultivating the virtue of civility. Daniel Bell defines *civitas* as "that spontaneous willingness to obey the law, to respect the rights of others, to forego the temptation of private enrichment at the expense of the public weal—in short, to honor the 'city' of which one is a member."[21] "Civility," Edward Shils writes, "is an attitude and a pattern of conduct. . . . It is an attitude of concern for the good of the entire society. It is solicitous of the well-being of the whole, or the larger interest."[22] According to the political theorists Jean Cohen and Andrew Arato,

> It is on this terrain that we learn how to compromise, take reflective distance from our own perspective so as to entertain others, learn to value difference, recognize or create anew what we have in common, and come to see which dimensions of our traditions are worth preserving and which ought to be abandoned or changed. . . . More fundamentally, civility is the conduct of a person whose individual self-consciousness has been partly superseded by his collective self-consciousness. . . . It is the readiness to moderate particular, individual, or parochial interests and to give precedence to the common good.[23]

It is through these personal interactions that we come to appreciate the dignity and moral worth of fellow community members. In civil society, people "become part of the world of family, friends, comrades, and colleagues, where people are connected to one another and made responsible for one another."[24]

If well-being is defined in terms of living more closely attuned to values that matter, one question immediately arises: "Matters to whom?" As Sandel charges, a defining characteristic of the modern era is the fear that any attempt to define the common good will interfere with the pursuit of individual self-interests.[25] But, rather than acquiescing to the priority of procedural protections (or seeing no alternative), we might consider the degree to which these fears may be an artifact of sociocultural conditions in which a sense of belongingness and the social practices that promote that identification and concern for the whole have disintegrated. Identification with the whole gives one a different perspective on potential constraints on the pursuit of individual self-interests. It makes possible a transition in self-understanding, from "I" to "we."

To the extent that we identify with larger social groups, we experience a metamorphosis in self-understanding. The boundaries of self-interests expand, opening onto expressions of "we" and "our interests" beyond "me" and "my interests." Seeing one's identity in terms of the roles and memberships of group affiliations—family, union, church, community, country, humanity—changes where we draw the line between self-interests and the interests of others, transforming concessions into common concerns. Sandel elaborates,

> One consequence of an enlarged self-understanding such as this is that when "my" assets or life prospects are enlisted in service of a common endeavor, I am likely to experience this less as a case of being used for others' ends and more as a way of

contributing to the purposes of the community I regard as my own. The justification of my sacrifice, if it can be called a sacrifice, is not the abstract assurance that unknown others will gain more than I will lose, but rather the more compelling notion that by my efforts I contribute to the realization of a way of life in which I take pride and with which my identity is bound.[26]

Through participation in social practices that promote civility, we redefine and expand the boundaries of social solidarity.

In addition to cultivating the virtue of civility, participation in civil society is essential for strengthening the faculty of practical reason. Since Aristotle's time, philosophers have recognized that there is no substitute for practice and experience in acquiring the capacity for good judgment. It is through public exchanges, debates, and deliberations that we become better at articulating and clarifying normative understandings about the meaning and value of different social practices. Do certain social practices help us to become better people, or do they make us more shallow, more fragmented, more depraved? Most people do not have ready-formed opinions about the wide range of issues that affect community life (such as the implications of introducing needle exchange programs or condom distribution programs in schools). Until people have the occasion to discuss a particular issue with others, their thoughts can be pretty vague and inchoate. We need to talk with others to push our thinking, to clarify and make more coherent the hazy jumble of half-baked, oft-confused considerations lying dormant in the recesses of our mind. It takes dialogue and debate to arrive at fuller understandings about the meanings of acts, and hence their evaluation.

Are needle exchange programs compassionate acts of reaching out to fellow human beings in an effort to prevent unnecessary suffering, or are they short-sighted, perhaps even dangerous, symbolic acts granting further license and legitimacy to hedonic, dissolute lifestyles? How we evaluate these practices depends on how we understand their meaning and purpose. To the extent that we can achieve public consensus that these programs are compassionate acts aimed at helping addicts put their lives back in order, then people will know that these programs do not abet drug abuse. If, instead, after deliberating, we see these programs as one more instance of telling ourselves that anything goes, that any and all behaviors are okay, and people can do whatever they feel like, then people may very well believe and act as though shooting heroin has been given the community's blessing. Normative understandings are forged in public forums and debates. It is in civil society that a more adequate expression of public opinion is formed.

Against this view, when the NIH researchers that we met in the first chapter deplore the intrusion of politics into the selection of strategies for AIDS prevention, they are seeking to preempt public discussions and remove decisions from the public domain.[27] The aim of saving lives is well-intentioned, but in asserting the authority of their office in order to trump the views of people who disagree with their means and ends, they do a disservice. Mandates backed by the power of office circumvent and impede the formation of public opinion. If heeded, the call would undercut the consolidation of public consensus about which norms are shared and binding. It is coming to these shared normative understandings that will ultimately make all the difference in how we, as a society, come to terms with issues like drug abuse and teen pregnancy.

Make no mistake, it is utopian to imagine any sweeping consensus of opinion. Real conflicts will persist. We will continue to disagree about the best way to live, about which values are more important than others, and about the contours of any programs to foster the good life. But, personally, I think this is what life is all about. In situations where there are conflicting conceptions of the good, it takes a refined, sensitive presence of mind to enable us to discern when claims about certain social practices should be judged either ill-conceived or deserving of support. There are no a priori procedural guarantees, no methods to invoke, that will insure that we make the correct decision. For health promotion professionals, the philosopher Hans Georg Gadamer has stated the challenge well: "In the end, this is the birth of the concept of reason: the more what is desirable is displayed for all in a way that is convincing to all, the more those involved discover themselves in this common reality; and to that extent human beings possess freedom in the positive sense, they have their true identity in that common reality."[28]

TRUST AND SOCIAL INTEGRITY

In this understanding, health promotion is the practice of bringing community members together to seek agreement on courses of action that will enhance the quality of shared community life. It is an ethical and political process of discussion, debate, and deliberation, in which ideas are convincing to the extent that people discover something of themselves and something of genuine value in their realization. It is the exercise of practical reason in civil society. But there are impediments to promoting this social practice. One of the most important barriers is the level of trust or mistrust in one's community. To wrap up this discussion, I want to propose that the level of trust shared by community members is an important indicator of the level of community well-being. High levels of trust are evidence of the fact that others will act with integrity in respecting values held in common. Low levels of trust (or high levels of mistrust) are indicative of situations in which people believe that others will unfairly seek to advance their own self-interests to the detriment of others.

Bernard Barber has identified three different meanings of trust. One is overarching and general; the other two are derivative of the first. The first and most general meaning of trust is the fulfillment of moral responsibility; the more specific meanings focus on technical competence and fiduciary obligation. Trust is characterized by expectations. As Barber states, "The most general is the expectation of the persistence and fulfillment of the natural and moral social orders."[29] In broad terms, trust is the expectation and general sense of confidence that others will not take unfair advantage of a situation to advance their own or their exclusive group interests. We trust others to carry out their promises, for example, despite opportunities to renege. We trust people to be honest, even when withholding information might be to their advantage. Under this broad umbrella, technical competence refers to the expectation that parties to particular types of interactions have the requisite skills and expertise to perform their roles effectively, as in "I trust my doctor will perform the operation well." Finally, fiduciary obligation refers to the institutional duty to place the interests of others before its own in situations such as trusteeships. It is the ethical obligation to make the concerns of others primary.

The sociologist Niklas Luhmann explains why trust is essential for the well-being of society.[30] Trust is crucial for reducing the complexity of social situations. In interactions in which trust is lacking, people are forced to assume that everyone else is strategically seeking to take advantage of the situation. As each person tries to anticipate the others' moves (to avoid getting the short end of the stick), the dynamic soon produces paralysis. Individuals become overburdened with the complexity of thinking about whether others will anticipate a response to their initial move, in which case they need to come up with a response to their response, and so on, into painfully taxing processes of wheel spinning. Trust, Luhmann contends, is the indispensable foundation for making decisions in situations where the consequences cannot entirely be anticipated. (In this vein, Francis Fukayama has recently made a provocative case for the idea that economic development is directly associated with the level of social trust within each nation–state, for all nations in the world.[31]) Without trust, social life would become unbearable. Indeed, the level of trust is indicative of the level of social well-being.

To the extent that public health promotion has concerned itself with the issue of trust, it has banked on perceptions of technical competence to convey its trustworthiness. For many public health issues, this is quite appropriate and public health has deservedly earned the trust of the public. Ensuring safe food and water supplies, mounting childhood immunization campaigns, and spearheading toxic waste cleanups depend on the skilled application of effective technologies. It is a different matter, however, with issues closer to the heart of health promotion, such as substance abuse, AIDS, smoking, teen pregnancy, and alcohol abuse. Here, the field urgently needs to reconsider current practices, in terms of both our technical competence and our fiduciary obligations.

Research attempting to identify generalizable causes of human behavior has not resulted in producing effective techniques to control or change human behavior, the kind of technical competence to which the scientific approach to health promotion aspires. There is now considerable public skepticism about the effectiveness of substance abuse, teen pregnancy, and other prevention programs in school settings, where conditions afford the most control over program implementation.[32] In less favorable conditions, the most carefully controlled community intervention trials, targeting smoking and heart disease prevention, for example, have likewise produced no significant results.[33] To continue to operate as if the field possessed the technical skills to produce social and behavioral change seems self-serving, and ultimately self-defeating. It undermines perceptions of our trustworthiness. Suggesting that health promotion specialists have (or are on their way to developing) the scientific expertise to solve the problems of infant mortality, substance abuse, and obesity is misleading. Community members quickly discover that we no better know our way out of the darkness than they. The inevitable disappointment lays bare a breach in trust founded on claims of such technical competence.

If fiduciary obligation is defined as the institutional obligation to put the interests of others ahead of its own, then public health practitioners face a paradox. Most people in the field are drawn to public health because of a sincere desire to serve the needs of others. Yet the imperatives of instrumental reason lead the field to define people's needs for them. To maximize efficiency, we know that heart disease is the leading cause of death, that smoking is the most significant risk factor, and, therefore, that community members must stop smoking. The field is not quite sure how to respond to expressions of concerns that have higher priority for community members. Because the logic of instrumental reason is almost irresistible, the field is put in an awkward position in such situations, proceeding as if community members were not fully cognizant or appreciative of their real interests. So, while on one level the field is putting its best understanding of the needs of others first, on another level many programs are perceived as engineered by elite professionals pursuing their own priorities regardless of the concerns expressed by community members.

The conduct of health promotion research faces similar problems and generates even greater strains since the purported benefits to others are further removed. The standard justification for conducting social scientific research is that the knowledge yielded will ultimately benefit society—not the participants themselves but others at some unknown point in the future. There are now open questions about such benefits. Many schools and communities refuse to be used any longer as "laboratories" for research. The jargon-larded prose of research write-ups as well as the mountains of trivial results are frequently lamented.[34] It is almost beyond imagination to think that community members might turn to reading professional journals to try to come to a better understanding of problems in their community. More telling, it is not clear if practitioners themselves find such research useful in trying to improve their practice.[35] The overwhelming impression is that the preponderance of research is produced because researchers face threats of "publish or perish" with respect to their career advancement. The bonds of trust are not strengthened by these practices. If we continue to seek power to effect changes in people's behavior, the likely result will be that we will continue to generate mistrust about our motives and about whose interests are being served.

The field of health promotion can do two things to foster greater trust in communities. First, the field needs to give up the illusion that a set of technical skills comparable to those of medical practitioners is on the horizon. We will never be able to control people's behavior in the way that we can now control microbes, and, more to the point, we should not want such control. We would be hard-pressed to call someone "well" whose conduct was determined by skilled interventions that produced targeted behavioral outcomes. We would think him instead a puppet or a robot. If one steps back and reflects on the kinds of goals most worth achieving, they would be quite the opposite of behavior control. We would want people to become the kinds of persons who are *not* driven by forces out of their control but who consciously choose and are responsible for their actions. To the extent that people's behavior is controlled or determined by external forces, a more worthy goal would be to liberate them from such forces. Health promotion professionals have much to offer in working with others to advance individual and community well-being, but not as behavioral scientists. They would do much better as public philosophers, creating a public space and reviving social practices through which we can all become more mindful of the kind of society we would like to live in together.

Second, we need to rethink our fiduciary obligations. This is a complex issue. I do not want to suggest that the expression of a particular concern by community members—or, as is more often the case, by some segment of the community—necessarily makes it the most important issue, for which we must drop all other considerations. But the field does need to become more truly collaborative in working with community members.

One major impediment is categorical funding. Most programs are funded to address one particular issue and do not now have the option of overriding that mandate. Institutionally, the field of public health should thus work toward expanding local control over the allocation of resources, moving away from categorical funding and toward block grants. There is already movement in this direction, for example, the new "federalism" of the national government. Expanding the sphere of local control is imminently feasible. Many programs are experimenting with community "mini-grant" initiatives and these could be expanded to good effect. Likewise, community development block grants have operated without predefined objectives for years. Expanding these types of programs will happen to the extent that we make it a priority, for reasons based at least in part on fulfilling our institutional fiduciary obligations. At the local level, the decision-making process could then be opened up, and indeed used as another opportunity for mutual reflection and deliberation over the best use of resources to promote the common good.

Furthermore, health promotion professionals frequently meet with church groups, unions, fraternities, social clubs, and neighborhood groups. In this alternative approach to health promotion, participation in these groups would no longer be conceived instrumentally, meeting with groups only to advance a strategic plan for changing their behavior. It would entail a shift in thinking about social participation, recast in terms of identity, belonging, and the bonds of community. Instead of using groups as a means of achieving predetermined objectives, health promotion should strive to create, maintain, and nurture public spaces that bring community members together to discuss matters of common concern. Interactions with community members in a non-instrumental, practical mode is based on identification and the realization of common values. In such relationships, we are equally likely to change our minds as we come to understand and appreciate their ideals regarding individual and community well-being.

The idea that community members should be given autonomy over program directions and the use of public health monies raises questions about accountability. Can grant or taxpayer dollars be allocated without defining in advance the outcomes to be achieved? How can program developers be held accountable if they do not specify exactly which problem will be addressed and how much progress they plan to accomplish before resources are awarded? I believe that programs can be fully accountable without usurping local authority by defining the targeted outcomes in advance. Instead of evaluating projects to see how they measure up in reaching the objectives defined in the project proposal, evaluation in this proposed alternative framework would focus on documenting what was accomplished, which could take many directions. This approach would also better suit the needs of community members. Currently, there is one program for tobacco education, one person assigned to AIDS education, and another one concerned with teen pregnancy prevention, all working with the same youth. The tobacco person does not talk about AIDS because it is outside the parameters of her funding stream. If she did, it would not fit on the monthly management information system (MIS) form nor count toward meeting her objectives.

Under new guidelines, these monies could be pooled, health promoters could work with community members to decide which issues are most important to address, and they would document all of the different activities and achievements that result. Taxpayers could then decide if they thought these activities were worthwhile and deserving of continued support. In the next chapter, we will learn about the work of one such program, El Centro de Educacion, Prevencion y Accion (CEPA, Center for Education, Prevention and Action). CEPA provides an excellent example of ongoing work in Holyoke that creates the space of civil society by bringing people together as equals and as fellow community members to decide which issues and which projects they want to undertake.

8

A NEW WAY OF PRACTICE

The distinguished professor of health education, Meredith Minkler, describes two competing traditions vying for the profession's allegiance. On the one hand, based on the specification of measurable objectives in the Surgeon General's *Healthy People 2000* report, Minkler notes the increasing tendency to focus on modifying individual behaviors. Consequently, "health promotion research and evaluation tend to become operationalized chiefly as the 'process of discovering alterable risk factors for [disease] and related strategies for eliminating or at least reducing these factors.'"[1] On the other hand, Minkler cites another stalwart tradition growing out of principles originally articulated by one of the early leaders in the field, Dorothy Nyswander. That tradition affirms unconditional respect for the dignity, integrity, and autonomy of individuals. In Dr. Nyswander's most famous words, health promotion must "start where the people are." In line with this heritage, Minkler defines health education as a process that fosters public participation, strengthens community and cultural identity, and enhances the quality of the physical and social environments.[2]

This chapter puts forth recommendations for alternative means of conducting research, professional education, and program design more consistent with the ends of health promotion developed in the preceding chapters. The challenge is how best to realign the institutional practices of health promotion to support this outlook on the sources of human well-being. What sorts of research activities would enable people to gain greater self-awareness and self-understanding? What types of research activities would enable people to develop their capacities for making more discerning judgments about matters of health and well-being? What sorts of academic training might better prepare public health promotion professionals for engaging with community members in deliberations about the good life and in collaborative efforts to create more decent and humane living conditions? What sorts of institutional practices would cultivate a disposition toward mindful, responsible choice? What sorts of programs might more conscientiously promote the pursuit of self-knowledge and inspire collective actions to work together to improve the quality of shared community life?

The three major institutional practices of health promotion—research, aining, and intervention programs—are tightly meshed. The purpose of research is to test hypotheses to determine the risk factors for ill health. After verifying their causal impact, programs are supposed to reduce or eliminate the identified risk factors so that unhealthy behaviors decrease and healthier behaviors increase. Public health professionals are schooled in the science of health promotion in academic training programs, learning which social–psychological theories and their associated interventions are most effective in producing targeted outcomes.

In an age that puts a premium on power and efficiency, letting go of the idea that health promotion is a science like medicine may put health education at a funding disadvantage, but it is ethically and epistemologically dubious to continue in the current direction. My proposal is to reorient research, training, and program activities toward strengthening people's capacity for reasoning wisely and cultivating greater mindfulness and civility, in practices that reintegrate means and ends. Rather than treating people as objects for study, my first recommendation is to engage in more participatory research, a process in which people come to understand themselves better and see more clearly what ought to be done to realize ends of their own choosing. Rather than instilling an ethos of technical efficiency, I recommend reorienting academic training programs to enhance students' capacities for exercising more discerning ethical and political judgment, wherein field work would necessarily assume greater prominence. Rather than having program objectives and methods prescribed by the results of experiments, we should break down the distinction between program developers and program recipients to the greatest extent possible, in a process in which health promoters would cast off the heavy mantle of behavior-change experts and rejoin their communities as fellow citizens.

RESEARCH FOR PRACTICAL PURPOSES

With the rise of the modern scientific outlook, research and theorizing about human behavior have become highly specialized. Theory must now take the form of statements from which testable hypotheses can be deduced. Thus, a typical definition from one of the better-known textbooks in the field describes theory as "a set of interrelated constructs (concepts), definitions, and propositions that present a systematic view of phenomena by specifying relations among variables, with the purpose of explaining and predicting the phenomena."[3] Successful prediction of the results of an experiment is the most rigorous test of the validity of theory. The dominant positivist paradigm thus runs directly counter to the idea that people are capable of self-knowledge and self-direction, appealing instead to the indispensability of scientific procedures for achieving valid knowledge and to the need for skilled expert interventions for disrupting the causal processes that result in unhealthy behaviors.

Two prospective directions for the field are now evident. Along one path, Glanz, Lewis, and Rimer present the orthodox view, "In health education and health behavior, as well as in this text, the dominant perspective that supports the largest body of theory and research is that of logical positivism."[4] Challenging this view, William Sullivan writes:

> The dimensions of the challenge [of resolving social problems] become clearer as we ask what stands in the way of an effective response. The answer is disturbing, though manifest. Beside, or rather behind, the inertia of entrenched interests there is also an ideal and a regime of knowledge which is strongly resistant to the stance of social engagement and moral inquiry demanded of today's challenges. This is the epistemic regime of positivism. . . . The continuing hold of positivistic dogma over the thinking and practice of higher education is a key problem which must be confronted by anyone who concludes that the needs of our time demand a reshaping of professional knowledge.[5]

Pointing a different direction, the sociologist Herbert Blumer defines theory in terms more consistent with the current needs of health promotion: "The point of developing theory is to outline and define life situations so that people may have a clearer understanding of their world through meaningful clarification of basic social values, modes of living, and social relations."[6]

The purpose of a reformed research agenda would be to promote self-knowledge and self-awareness and to refine our mutual capabilities for exercising more astute judgment about the kinds of values and principles we want to uphold. Fortunately, a model for this type of research already exists. Because of the shift in the nature of most modern health problems, research in health promotion must now go beyond positivism to incorporate the types of scholarly activities characteristic of research conducted in the humanities, such as the research and theorizing done in history, law, literature, and philosophy.[7]

Suppose that research did not necessarily have to be directed at formulating and testing hypotheses. Suppose that we acknowledged there were other equally valid forms of research and theorizing and that our colleagues in the humanities are just as committed to uncovering truths about the human condition as scientists are. How else might we think about the purposes of research in health promotion? What else might we seek to accomplish in conducting research? I will describe five purposes that theory and research could serve besides the positivist sine-qua-non pillars of prediction and explanation: (*1*) making assumptions explicit; (*2*) understanding; (*3*) sense-making; (*4*) sensitization; and, (*5*) critique. All offer different ways of clarifying values and of establishing the grounds for making such claims.

Participatory research[8] is the most logical approach to future research in health promotion, although, because of their institutional resources, academically based researchers have both greater opportunity and greater responsibility for initiating, carrying the workload, and writing up the results of research activities. In this vein, researchers and community members would act as co-investigators. This type of research is much more self-consciously and deliberately reflexive; it aims for achieving mutual understanding, in which both parties would be equal teachers and learners. It is a dialogical process in which academically trained researchers have a responsibility for bringing to the discussion reflections and insights from the scholarly literature, for what they are worth.[9] The test of the validity of this type of research is whether or not community members and researchers alike learn something about themselves such that they can live lives of greater integrity. As Lindblom notes, it is the difference between striving for a "scientific society" versus a "self-guiding" society.[10]

Making Assumptions Explicit

To highlight the differences between these two basic research orientations, I will start with an example that can be construed in either positivistic or humanistic terms.

When colleagues lament the gap between theory and practice today, they are referring to the common observation that practitioners rarely design programs based explicitly on any of the field's familiar theories.[11] More often than not, practitioners call on their experience and common sense in developing programs. How might the two different frameworks for research bridge this gap? One potential purpose of theorizing is to make assumptions explicit.

A popular exercise in youth development programs these days is to draw a "life map," a picture of major life events from birth onwards. If one were to look for an explicit theoretical basis for this exercise, like Social Learning Theory, the Theory of Protection Motivation, or the Transtheoretical Model, none would be found. But if one were to ask the practitioner why she decided to conduct this exercise, a wealth of ideas would inevitably emerge. The exercise builds trust, which may be lacking in these youths' lives. It creates an open atmosphere, a space where they can feel safe to disclose problems that are bothering them. It is cathartic— the opportunity to talk about problems in and of itself releases some of the pain the young people are carrying. It is fun and engaging, engrossing otherwise bored youth. Behind each of these ideas are implicit notions about why young people get into trouble these days: they are isolated, with no one they can trust or turn to for support, they have been hurt, they are bored.

From a positivist perspective, each of these ideas needs to be transformed into hypotheses for testing to determine their validity. Researchers should strive to develop operational definitions to measure social isolation, painful life events, and boredom, and then look for correlations with identified public health problems, such as substance abuse or unprotected sex. If they find a correlation, then the most powerful test of the validity of these factors is to conduct an experiment, with random assignment to treatment and control groups. An intervention (perhaps something like the life map exercise) is conducted to see if it lowers the treatment group's sense of isolation, desolation, boredom, etc., and then one observes whether these changes lead to reductions in problem behaviors. Only after conducting these experiments would the field know for sure that boredom, etc., are valid risk factors that should be targeted for intervention.

But a more humanistic outlook suggests a different approach. From a humanistic perspective, the causal significance of these factors pales before their significance in terms of meaningfulness.[12] Boredom does not cause youth to do anything. It is a feeling and a way of experiencing the moment about which one may choose to do something or not. It may mean one needs to learn to recognize, name, and deal with the discomfort. It may mean it is time to take up a hobby. Or it may require only an act of reinterpretation, as in enjoying the pleasures of idle summer days.[13]

From the positivist perspective, the condition is viewed instrumentally, as a risk factor, something to be reduced or eliminated in order to solve health and social problems. But from a humanistic perspective, these experiences are the warp and woof of people's lives. How we think about them (e.g., boredom as threatening risk factor versus boredom as time free of demands) molds the experience, and hence the range of potential responses. The experience of boredom raises questions: about the degree to which life should be filled with constant stimulation and distractions; about how much we should demand of ourselves and others that these times be devoted to constructive, elevating uses; about the shape of the life that we want to live as all of us grope for ways to make good use of our spare time. Researchers can point out the problematic issues, raising questions for discussion and deliberation to which all parties can be invited to respond. Striving to identify and make open and apparent the unspoken premises of an exercise, and hence one's speculations about what makes people tick, creates an opportunity to open up a dialogue about formerly implicit, unexamined presumptions about the reasons people do things like turn to drugs. Together, people can decide whether they want to do something about the situation or not.

For researchers, a change in perspective has many implications. Rather than regarding practitioners as either ignorant or negligent about the utility of proven theories, researchers could come to see practitioners as primary resources for stimulating their thinking and theorizing. Rather than trying to come up with a single standardized operational definition of an experience (such as feeling bored), researchers could seek out as many facets and dimensions as possible of the ways in which people perceive these subjective states, trying to uncover the full gamut of rich and variegated descriptions that explore all the nuances, shades of meaning, and paradoxes in their experience. Such studies would help practitioners, researchers, and community members alike become more articulate about their own assumptions and better able to recognize when they are having trouble making their own assumptions more explicit.

Understanding

After prediction and explanation, the most frequently nominated purpose of theorizing is understanding. Extensive discussions of the differences between explanation and understanding have been put forward elsewhere, as in Von Wright's *Explanation and Understanding* and Apel's *Understanding and Explanation*. Where explanation seeks to make events predictable through knowledge of causes, understanding seeks to make phenomena intelligible through knowledge of their *telos*: their aim, intention, purpose, and meaning.[14]

The inclusion of understanding would expand the boundaries of research to include not only the search for causes of behavior, but also the task of grasping its underlying rationale, its meaning, morality, and motivation.[15] From a humanistic perspective, the search for independent, antecedent causes will never be sufficient to explain behavior because a more complete understanding depends on comprehending the aims, purposes, and intentions of the individual. While intentions are influenced by past events, they take shape mainly in a creative process of picturing how one would like to exercise one's agency, one's will, to change the course of future events. They are unpredictable precisely to the degree that decisions are informed by the unique features of the particular situation, individual interpretations of the meaning that events hold for them, and the human capacity to exercise free choice about how one ought to live.[16] To understand people's behavior, researchers must look beyond prior causes to search for its meaning and intent. These meanings are expressed as reasons for the choice of one course of action over another.

Theory as understanding is often presented in the form of narratives, the most common way humans organize experience to comprehend its meaning.[17] As MacIntyre states, "We always move toward placing a particular episode in the context of a set of narrative histories. . . . In what does the unity of an individual life consist? The answer is that its unity is the unity of a narrative embodied in a single life. . . . I can only answer the question, 'What am I to do?' if I can answer the prior question 'Of what story do I find myself a part?'"[18] The value and validity of this type of theorizing are experienced as revelation—the "ah-ha" experience, as in "now I get it, now I understand why they chose that course of action."

If this type of theorizing were more widely accepted and available in the field, community members and practitioners could turn to research not for prescriptions about what to do, but for insight into their own lives.[19] If theory and research were not limited to developing and testing hypotheses, we could better appreciate the value of reading, for example, a historical description of the role of individualism in American life, as provided by Bellah and his colleagues in their masterful *Habits of the Heart* (1985). The value of this type of research comes not from drawing conclusions about whether individualism is a risk factor that needs to be eliminated, but from seeing more clearly the ways in which we may unconsciously and unintentionally reinforce this value and from recognizing its many permutations better as we struggle to figure out what is going on in our society. In my research, for example, I tried to apply the theoretical insights gleaned from Bellah's account to gain a better understanding of recurrent cycles of substance abuse throughout American history, with the aim of illuminating current trends.[20] Through this type of historical research and theorizing, features of situations that were formerly opaque, puzzling, or obscured are made more salient and recognizable.

Sense-Making

Another function of theorizing is "sense-making." The distinction from the above is that "understanding" is generally considered a process of discovery, whereas "sense-making" acknowledges the conscious act of creation, the human mind actively imposing order on the chaos of sense perceptions.[21]

The sense-making function of theory introduces the notion of the social construction of reality,[22] or as Searle emended the phrase, the construction of social reality.[23] The claim here is that, in the social world, the ethical principles and values by which we lead our lives are not located in the structure of the universe waiting to be discovered, but rather they are corrigible products of the human creative mind and hence subject to constant revision and reformulation as we try to make better sense of how we should live. As theory is used here, researchers do not deny that explicating a situation is a creative act in which the researcher—with "values, warts, and all"[24]—actively molds how events are to be interpreted. The process of developing theory is more one of making rather than finding, creating rather than uncovering.[25] As Anderson notes, researchers are "not discovering meaning but bravely imputing meaning to a universe, which, more likely than not, has none."[26] Theory is often presented in the form of a descriptive diagnosis of a situation.

An example from my own work illustrates the application of this type of theorizing to health promotion. In a case study of community coalition building, I was struggling to make sense of the constant tensions and frequent breakdowns in communication between community members and university academics.[27] Using the community organizing typology developed by Rothman,[28] I thought it might be helpful if people saw how the actions of community members could be interpreted in terms of the principles of "locality development," whereas the actions of academics were better described in terms of an expert "social planning" approach. The analysis enabled us to see that community members and academics might come to the table with different goals, assumptions, basic change strategies, etc., in mind. Thus, we could better see how and why the two parties frequently talked past one another, failed to see the significance of issues voiced by the other side, and failed to understand why the others did not share their concerns.

There is no claim to have discovered that community members are innately "locality developers" or academics "social planners" in a way that leads them invariably to act in certain ways. The point of this type of theorizing is to help those involved (and readers of the write-up) get a handle on potential sources of confusion and frustration. It gives people points of reference for a discussion to see if they can work out their differences. The test of its validity is whether it does, in practice, help people make sense of their situation.

Sensitization

The sensitizing function of theory aims to heighten people's awareness of the broadest possible range of contingencies bearing on a specific situation. In contrast to the search for generalizable factors, theory and research are here used to sharpen, highlight, and bring to the foreground as many aspects as possible that make the situation under investigation unique and different from other situations.

Blumer suggests that the way researchers "outline life situations" is through identifying "sensitizing concepts."[29] Examples of this type of theorizing are the analytic themes and ideal types that emerge in ethnographies, field work, case studies, and the like. The anthropologist Clifford Geertz's call for "thick description" likewise speaks to this function of theorizing.[30]

An example of a sensitizing concept is the theoretical construct of "institutional embeddedness."[31] Through in-depth interviews, I found that some youth frame decisions about drug use in terms of their roles within their families, schools, church, and community (e.g., "I'm Baptist and Baptists are not allowed," "I couldn't do drugs, it would let the team down"), whereas others think about the decision in terms of individual desires (e.g., "I don't feel like it"). There is a distinct structure to their respective perceptions (embedded or not) about what is relevant to the decision. Through these types of studies we become more sensitive to what is going on in a situation; without them, certain features would pass unnoticed.

The value of such studies is that people can develop a more perceptive, more discerning appreciation of their unique circumstances when they have these concepts available to them. When one reads a good (precise, authentic, accurate, persuasive[32]) case study, aspects of a situation about which one was formerly blind become more apparent. The warrants for the validity of these theoretical constructs are the felt capacities of users for acting more lucidly/less blindly, more cognizantly/less obliviously, with a keener, more refined sense of discrimination.

Critique

The final purpose of research presented here is critique. Gitlin recalls that social theory was historically conceived as social criticism in service of social change.[33] Theory as critique traces its roots to the emancipatory project of the Enlightenment, particularly as it focused on the problems arising from existing power structures.[34] Sociology began as an attempt to find footing for social critique. If one thinks of the works of Marx, Durkheim, or Weber, all were deeply concerned about the contemporary state of society. Each in his own way was trying to flesh out ideas for alternative forms of social organization as a way of calling attention to problems in his society.

The purpose of theorizing as critique is to challenge a going concern by holding it up to a more ideal image.[35] This form of theorizing confronts the status quo by asking questions that need to be asked, raising issues that need to be raised, and spelling out alternatives to claims about the inevitability of existing conditions. In its most provocative form, researchers in this mode write about piercing the veil of ideological hegemony to root out false consciousness. In its less strident forms, theory as critique is an effort to rethink accepted doctrine by postulating different possible futures. The best known critical theorist in health education is the Brazilian educator Paolo Freire.[36] While the decline of this type of theorizing has been lamented,[37] the tradition lives on in numerous works, such as Bellah, et al's., *The Good Society* (1991) and Gitlan's *The Twilight of Common Dreams* (1995).

Caveats

Before concluding this section, two points that continue to bedevil the field need to be addressed. First, there is a misunderstanding that the alternative to positivist research methodologies is "qualitative" research. Qualitative research per se is not the corrective proposed here. On the one hand, qualitative studies do not necessarily challenge the aims and assumptions of the positivist program of research; often, they are subsumed as exploratory or hypothesis-generating research. As we saw in Chapter 2, such research is considered a normal first step in a process that culminates in the true test of the validity of a proposition: randomized control trials. On the other hand, if by qualitative research one means studies that are opposed to counting observations, that is not the kind of research recommended here either. Research can be empirical and it can quantify observations without subscribing to the tenet that truth can only be determined by making successful predictions.

But there is another sense in which qualitative research, more broadly understood, *is* the proposed corrective. This is usually referred to as interpretive, or hermeneutic, research. The need for interpretive research arises because values are not strictly empirical. Values such as justice, equality, dignity, or well-being do not lend themselves to strict operational definition. They do not fit neatly into operational definitions because they are not "things" with fixed empirical referents. Rather, they are evolving ideals about how we think we ought to live. As research shifts increasingly toward clarifying basic social values, there will be a corresponding need for using more interpretive approaches and in exercising greater caution before forcing operational definitions on ideas that inexorably entail qualitative discriminations of worth. In the framework recommended here, however, such interpretive studies would no longer be viewed as preliminary, epistemologically inferior research, but rather that which is most sorely needed in the field today.

There is also much misunderstanding about the meaning and implications of the term "postmodernism." To the extent that "postmodern" means one no longer believes in the Enlightenment dream that all questions have one and only one true answer, that there is one and only one method to arrive at this truth, and that all these truths will be compatible with one another once uncovered,[38] then this book is certainly postmodern. But once these Enlightenment assumptions were called into question, some people have gone on to claim that the whole idea of science is a charade, and even more strongly, that truths of any nature cannot be established at all, reducing all such attempts to "language games" and discourses of power.[39] That is not a position I share. Experimental science works perfectly well in many fields. We can even learn things from quasi-experimental designs in the social sciences on occasion, particularly in trying to determine whether changes in policies or programs produce their intended results, although I still think far too much stock is put in this trade. The processes of change (or factors accounting for the lack of change) and the range of outcomes are usually too diffuse for the relatively insensitive instruments typically used in social studies.

Finally, against other points of view,[40] I think that there are grounds for establishing truths about the human condition that lie in successful communication.[41] It is possible for people to reach reasoned, nonarbitrary, noncoerced agreement— to seek out and achieve common understandings—about the kinds of lives and the kinds of societies that are good for human beings. These understandings are true, even if we may later change our minds.

In sum, I think that testing hypotheses in the social domain is epistemologically and ethically dubious, the high value placed on identifying generalizable factors misguided, and the investment in operational definitions damaging to human sensibilities. A change in perspective would enable us to incorporate the observations and reflections of other fields, such as literature, history, and philosophy, breaking down the unwholesome barriers that have arisen between the humanities and the social sciences. By moving back and forth between empirical observations and philosophical analyses, creative portrayals, and historical accounts, research reports could provide the kind of knowledge that would help community members arrive at new insights, offer new ways of looking at an issue, and bring new food for thought in public discussions.

It has always struck me as odd that the current approach to social scientific research has put such stock in the replication and convergence of results, where the humanities value developing new insights and new interpretations. Boyle's Law has stayed essentially the same since its original formulation in the seventeenth century. Every year, hundreds of new interpretations and new insights into the works of Shakespeare are produced. The Health Belief Model, Social Learning Theory, and the Theory of Reasoned Action have stayed essentially the same since their original formulation in the 1950s. If the model of the natural sciences is correct, the goal of social research is to discover analogous models of human behavior that are eternally and universally true. If, however, the model of humanistic research is more befitting, then we might come to appreciate the prospect of each new study revealing new insights.

In conclusion, the field of health promotion needs the kind of research that can help all of us—researchers, practitioners, and community members alike—become more sensitive, critical, articulate, constructive, less oblivious to subtle social dynamics, less blind to unconscious assumptions, and more understanding of the complexities of modern life. This research could profitably take three new directions.

First, academically based researchers need to work more closely with practitioners and community members, but turning the tables to see what researchers can learn from them, rather than telling them which hypotheses one plans to test. What are the implicit theories practitioners are putting into practice? Such research is dialogical, going back and forth, give and take, as all parties struggle to articulate tacit assumptions and make sense of the swirl of events whenever one engages in the struggle to improve social conditions. Second, researchers need to write up more case studies, ethnographies, field work, historical reconstructions, thought pieces, analyses of themes from focus groups, oral histories, key informant interviews, policy analyses, critiques, and voices of public opinion. Third, public health education researchers need to actively incorporate the work of scholars in philosophy, history, and literature in reflecting about ways to build a better world.

In this mode, the real test of the value and validity of health promotion theories would lie in their ability to inspire discussion, self-understanding, and action. Supported by research of this kind, community members would participate directly in deciding which questions to ask and in assessing which answers make sense to them. Supported by such research, practitioners could make public health truly public, raising questions for all concerned community members to deliberate. The value of this type of research grows out of the opportunity to help each other see things in a new light so that all of us might experience moral growth. Ultimately, the success of this approach would be seen in the flourishing of people's capacity to discern excellence from nonsense, to judge good from bad ideas, and to rectify efforts to live together decently.

PROFESSIONAL PREPARATION

Over the past 30 years, the National Commission for Health Education Credentialing and the two most prominent national professional associations, the Society for Public Health Education and the American Association for Health Education, have invested considerable energies in defining the professional skill competencies expected of qualified health promotion practitioners. The updated and revised 1997 standards define competencies in 10 skill areas: conducting needs assessments; planning and implementing effective health education programs; evaluation; coordination; acting as an information resource; communication; research methods; administration; and advancing the profession.[42] The application of behavioral science theory is identified as an essential subcompetency in 8 out of the 10 skill areas.

The revised 1997 standards include several new subcompetencies. Under Advancing the Profession, one of these is the application of ethical principles. Specified subcompetencies here include the ability to: (1) "analyze the interrelationships among ethics, values, and behavior;" (2) "relate the importance of a code of ethics to professional practice;" and, (3) "subscribe to a professionally recognized health education code of ethics."[43]

Academic programs are designed to impart these skills. To secure national accreditation, academic programs must demonstrate strong linkages between required courses and the national standards defining the field's professional skills. Such requirements typically include courses in behavioral science theory, needs assessment, program planning, program evaluation, group dynamics, and research methods.

In 1988, the National Academy of Sciences issued an alarmed report, *The Future of Public Health*, decrying a state of "disarray" in the field and observing that schools of public health had "become somewhat isolated"[44] from the practice of public health. The report recommended establishing closer affiliations between academia and practitioners. The influence of these recommendations is evident in the revised 1995 guidelines for accreditation issued by the Council on Education in Public Health (CEPH), with a pronounced emphasis on demonstrating collaborative ties between schools of public health and state and local health departments. In response, schools of public health have moved in the direction of making field work a more integral part of professional preparation. Still, requirements for field work are grossly uneven across program tracks within schools and across the 27 accredited schools of public health in the country. What are we to make of this change in training programs?

In *Work and Integrity: The Crisis and Promise of Professionalism in America*, William Sullivan traces the evolution in understanding what it means to be a professional in modern America:

> The most constant tension has been between a technical emphasis which stresses specialization—broadly linked to a utilitarian conception of society as a project for enhancing efficiency and individual satisfaction—and a sense of professional mission which has insisted upon the prominence of the ethical and civic dimensions of the enterprise. . . . This [latter understanding] is a tradition which, while acknowledging the genuine importance of technical proficiency in every field, views the professional enterprise as humanly engaged practices which generate values of great significance for modern societies.[45]

Sullivan characterizes the two poles as the difference between careers versus callings. "This distinction rests in part upon the institutional differentiation between the processes of markets and technological production which are guided by the criteria of instrumental efficiency, on the one hand, and the human activities organized in civil society, on the other hand, which aim at very different goals, such as moral agreement or cultural consensus."[46]

As careers, professions offer many rewards. Professionals acquire prized, extraordinary skills. They have unparalleled autonomy in defining their working conditions. They hold prestigious social positions (although their reputation has become somewhat tarnished of late). They are well compensated for their services. In return, they promise to provide the most effective and efficient ministrations possible. At the other end of the spectrum, Sullivan examines the historical roots of understanding professions as callings: "The term profession is itself religious in origin. It derives from the act of commitment, the declaration to enter on a distinct way of life, as in the profession of monastic vows. It was, at least in theory, a response to a belief that one had received a 'call,' not an action imposed by economic or other necessity. Profession entailed a commitment to embody the virtues needed to realize the community's highest purposes."[47]

Entering a profession was thought to be the fruit of conversion, of having been given a special task, and thus, of finding one's place in life.[48] To become a professional meant to commit one's life to a mission, understood as a sacred trust to promote and to act for the sake of declared common purposes.[49] Sullivan cites Jane Addams and her work at Hull House as the apotheosis of professionalism linked to this broader vision of generating trust and active social participation among citizens.[50] Sullivan's fear is that this older sense of civil service, oriented toward care for the moral and political integration of social life, has been overshadowed by a modern, more narrowly technical understanding.[51] As the revised standards for the public health education profession demonstrate, his concerns appear well-founded.

To recover and strengthen the profession's ethical and civic dimensions, five changes are recommended. First, the curriculum needs to be reconstructed to incorporate research of the type described above. As in law school curricula, many courses could be better organized around case studies through which students can enhance their capacity for exercising discerning judgment. Rather than learning sets of variables from select theories of human behavior to be used in defining operational program objectives, students need intensive practice in examining morally complex situations in order to apprehend more clearly the good and bad parts in actual community programs. What commends what they did? How might it be improved? How would you do things differently? Why? What are good reasons for proposing another line of action? What is worth preserving? It is a pragmatic, problem-centered approach that draws on the experiences of all involved in a process of refining sensibilities through discussion and reflection.

Second, the curriculum could be improved by incorporating historical investigations. Currently, students are not required to know anything about the history of the field; rarely are they even offered the option. This makes sense against a backdrop that presupposes the subject matter is composed of eternal, universal, scientific truth. In medicine, it is irrelevant how the ancient Greeks thought about human physiology. But is the same true of the social sciences? According to the philosopher Bernard Williams, "Human conventions . . . can be understood only with the help of history, and the social sciences accordingly have an essential historical base."[52] We need a historical perspective to understand the major issues now facing the field. The history of health promotion is replete with the rise and fall of periodic health crusades, proud accomplishments and quirky fads.[53] Entering professionals would be well served by reviewing this history, thereby gaining a critical perspective on current trends and their own motives for entering the field.

Third, the field needs to pay greater attention to its ethical foundations. In a recent survey, only 1 out of 24 schools required ethics instruction for all students.[54] Generally, these courses focus on a specific subcategory of ethics called bio-ethics. It is usually an elective and structured around what is sometimes referred to as "lifeboat" or quandary ethics.[55] In this type of course, students examine a series of topics that present moral dilemmas: Should a mother abort a fetus with a horrible genetic defect? Should a hopelessly terminally ill patient's life support system be turned off? Should alcoholics be excluded as candidates for liver transplants? In the glow of the Enlightenment dream, this type of modern ethical inquiry proceeds on the faith that with due perseverance one overriding ethical principle will eventually emerge in the analysis. Many philosophers are now skeptical of the notion that we will someday come up with one single coherent system of hierarchically ranked principles to which everyone subscribes, no matter how long we ponder these tragic dilemmas.[56] While there is some benefit to this type of discussion, I am more concerned about providing incoming professionals with sufficient grounding in moral philosophy to stimulate their capacity for recognizing and articulating the tacit ethical assumptions underlying various social theories, health promotion programs, and public debates[57] today. To this end, they might be better served by courses that introduce the history of ethics, the resurgence of virtue ethics,[58] and current debates about the relationship between the right and the good. "Practical social scientists," Bellah asserts, "are necessarily also philosophers, particularly moral philosophers, and should be familiar with the history of ethical thought."[59]

Fourth, programs need to think more self-consciously about processes of mentoring, both within and outside the school. Many faculty members are reluctant to think of themselves as role models, but most schools are also blessed with one or two professors whose experience, integrity, and bearing make them widely admired. Students need access and exposure to the thinking and composure of those who inspire us to fulfill the profession's highest callings. Outside the school, programs now put great emphasis on the professional credentials of field placement supervisors. If the aim of the alternative recommended here is to enhance people's capacity for practical judgment, the criteria for selecting preceptors might be broadened to good effect.

Finally, field work. There has been more emphasis placed on field experience since the publication of *The Future of Public Health* report, but the rationale has never been quite clear. Internships, where they are offered, are frequently fit into curricula as an afterthought or an appendage to come into compliance with accreditation standards, certainly not because they are considered the cornerstone of professional education. There is a vague hope that field work will somehow bridge the gap between theory and practice, providing students an opportunity to test out their newly acquired technical skills. In this context, one often hears communities referred to as "learning laboratories." But these grounds prove slim indeed, as the disjunction between the challenges of coming to terms with modern malaise and the illusions of technical prowess becomes more evident during the course of field practice. As one mentor observed, "It's politics. You know, everything they never teach you in school."

There are strong foundations justifying the value of field work, but they lie not in the mastery of technical skills. Sullivan comments that the need for institutional reform "also suggests a professional education in which practice is recognized as a potential source of knowledge and cultivated as such rather than relegated to second-rate status as simply an application of independently derived theory."[60] Field work is crucial because insight comes of experience. Judgment gets better over time with regular practice. Seasoning is crucial in strengthening and refining the faculty of practical reason.

PROGRAMS AS PUBLIC SPACES
FOR ENGAGING COMMUNITY

The pioneering heart disease prevention programs, such as the Stanford Three- and Five-Community studies, the North Karelia project, the Minnesota Heart Health plan and the Pawtucket, RI project,[61] are famous examples of the scientific approach to health promotion. The CEPA project provides a case study of the possibilities for engaging in an alternative mode of practice.

Because of mounting dissatisfactions with expert interventions, the W. K. Kellogg Foundation initiated the Community-Based Public Health (CBPH) program in March 1991.[62] In Holyoke, El Centro de Educacion, Prevencion, y Educacion CEPA was started under the auspices of the CBPH initiative.[63] Six years after its inception, CEPA now operates under the direction of its coordinator, Carmen Claudio, and an Advisory Board composed of local community members.

Soon after Kellogg announced the initiative, I met with and later joined the Holyoke Latino Community Coalition (HLCC) to seek their collaboration in this effort. They agreed. During the first year of the Community-Based Public Health initiative, we initiated a process for identifying priority issues and concerns in the community. One major advantage of the CBPH initiative was that there were no preconceived notions about the types of public health problems to be addressed. This structure enabled the coalition to pursue whichever community priorities emerged rather than starting with predefined goals (like the federal heart disease prevention programs) or with restrictions tied to categorical funding typically found in most grant initiatives today.

A group of HLCC members began gathering information about community priorities through small group discussions, individual interviews, and a community-wide public forum. The responses gathered in these discussions shed light on people's perceptions of community needs. They illustrate the differences between community-centered research and standardized scientific needs assessments (such as the CDC's Behavioral Risk Factor Survey). We asked community members, "¿Que cosas necesitan las personas/comunidades para ser saludables?" ("What do people/communities need to be healthy?"). In addition to things like food and jobs, more intangible responses included "a person you can trust," "leaders who care," "role models," "purpose in life," "a sense of moral coherence," "good relationships," and "a good basis for spiritual growth."

From these community discussions, the coalition proposed to initiate an HIV/ AIDS prevention program called CEPA ("cepa" can be translated as "core" or "root," as in family roots in genealogical trees). The fundamental philosophy of the CEPA project is to break down the distinction between program developers and program recipients to the greatest degree possible. The staff recruits neighborhood residents to meet and discuss what can be done about AIDS in Holyoke. The purpose of these discussions is to gain a clearer, more explicit, more self-conscious understanding of the difficulties community members face in protecting themselves from exposure to the virus.

CEPA staffs a storefront office in the Flats, a distressed neighborhood with rundown housing stock, high unemployment rates, and high numbers of school drop-outs, sex industry workers, drug dealers, and shooting galleries. In the core work of CEPA, the coordinator Carmen Claudio and two outreach workers go door-to-door, stand out on street corners, and call on various social organizations, church groups, tenant associations, community agencies, and any other establishments that bring people together. They introduce themselves, talk about what CEPA is trying to do, and invite neighborhood residents to join them in discussions about what can be done to prevent AIDS and improve community life in Holyoke. Over the years, the CEPA staff members have learned that building trust is a slow process. The trust and regard residents have for CEPA has grown as people have come to recognize that the staff respects them and treats them as fellow community members with whom they share much in common, not as clients to be treated.

CEPA tries to recruit 10–20 neighborhood residents for each round of discussions. After recruiting residents, the community members meet once a week for 2 hours in the evening to partake in structured discussions that go on over a 3-month period. The weekly meetings, in which staff and coalition members also participate, are conducted as a process of collective consciousness-raising. Using case studies and narratives as stepping off points for discussion, the sessions let participants identify the needs, barriers, and resources they personally experience in coping with threats to their health and well-being, including AIDS.

A framework guiding these discussions was developed based on philosophies of empowerment and participatory education. Drawing on the work of Paolo Freire, Wallerstein describes the empowerment process as consisting of listening, dialogue, problem-posing, and action.[64] As we discovered, however, the respective models (empowerment and participatory education) are not entirely compatible. In the empowerment model, there is a tendency toward locating the root causes of health problems in an unjust social structure, while in models of participatory education, the analysis draws on people's experiences and is consequently more open about where the analysis might lead.[65]

As the sessions progress, the discussions increasingly focus on identifying activities that will help people respond to the presence of AIDS in their neighborhood. The kinds of actions that community members think valuable are then framed as simple, user-friendly "requests for proposals." For example, one group decided that neighborhood efforts should focus on the teenage population with four major goals: (1) to promote self-esteem and self-determination, both individually and collectively; (2) to promote life-enhancing family values; (3) to create a public space for the Puerto Rican community; and, (4) to foster better communication, especially within families. The point, as one participant put it, is that "You have to feel pretty good about yourself to want to protect yourself from HIV."

In the next stage, to extend community involvement, a call for action is issued through the requests for proposals, providing financial support up to $5000. The proposals are circulated in the community through flyers, radio announcements, newspaper articles, outreach, handbills, mailings, community parties, presentations in agencies, press conferences, open houses, and word of mouth.

With on-going support from CEPA staff and modest financial resources (typically $2000–$3000), groups who respond, usually drawn together around a church or neighborhood group, set out to do what they can to improve community life. Examples include a teen drop-in center (submitted and run by teenagers), community forums, improvisational theater, park clean-ups, recreational activities, and a group of mothers (Grupo Educadores Latinas in Accion [GELA]) who set up dance, music, and basketball lessons for neighborhood teens. CEPA has also opened a neighborhood drop-in center for drug addicts.

These projects nurture a web of community relationships. The CEPA staff have a radically different understanding of their relationship to neighborhood residents. It is based on caring and friendship, not professional expert–client interactions. CEPA has maintained relationships with groups of residents for more than 5 years, (and counting), replenishing a reservoir of mutual trust and interdependence in the community. Staff live in the neighborhood; together it is their shared community life they want to enhance.

How do people find value in life? How do we nurture caring, commitment, and concern for the world around us? CEPA starts by asking people what they think would be worthwhile to do for their community. What do they think is important? What do they care about enough to want to commit their time and energy? Emerging from dialogue, these small resident-identified and resident-run projects try to reconnect people with what they see as valuable in this life, to become more mindful of what matters, here and now, where they find themselves, in the concrete particulars of this neighborhood, with these neighbors, homes and local history. In their work in Holyoke, the CEPA staff members identify and join with fellow community members in the struggle to ward off despair, alienation, and meaninglessness. If people can find something of value in their circumstances of life, they have reason to think about what they are doing, to weigh their options.

At this point in the history of CEPA, both the benefits of engaging with the community and the difficulties of living up to such an ideal are becoming clearer. The dilemmas of encouraging community members to define their own goals and methods in the face of many conflicting forces and contrary expectations have become a central theme in ongoing discussions. These discussions are illustrative of the exercise of practical reason where judgments are based on insight into particular circumstances.

From the outset, the coalition has wrestled with questions about how to define the project. We were committed to a process of engaging community members in defining the ends and means of CEPA, but funding agencies typically require highly specific delineation of program objectives and methods before allocating support. How then are we supposed to specify the program goals and activities before engaging the very people who are to decide which are most appropriate?

In the original grant proposal, we settled on a painstaking compromise that described the participatory community involvement process but also listed a number of possible goals and activities. The W. K. Kellogg Foundation accepted the idea. But when CEPA has sought additional funding, other grant agencies have responded as expected in demanding to know the specific, targeted objectives for which resources were being requested. It has been difficult to obtain support for the idea that program objectives and methods would emerge from the process and could take many unforeseeable forms.

We pondered the composition of the resident groups. After lengthy discussions, we decided to engage as diverse a group of community members as possible rather than seek specific subgroups (such as sex workers or adolescents). In contrast to social marketing theories proclaiming the effectiveness of market segmentation, we thought the idea of recruiting community residents according to specified target categories would further fragment the community by emphasizing differences over more significant, shared commonalties.

We had to decide whether to pay participants or not. We weighed whether external monetary rewards would detract from a spirit of *civitas* and voluntary giving to the community. We looked at the poverty statistics. After reflecting on the alternatives, we decided to give residents stipends for their participation, agreeing that financial compensation was due for their time, knowledge, and labor.

In deciding about the structure of the discussions, we again wrestled with the trade-offs. If the sessions were plotted beforehand, then we would be imposing control, setting up an operation that tells participants what we expect them to consider important, and inevitably reproducing our own assumptions, interests, and biases. But if we did not provide any structure to the discussions, people might think we were unprepared and did not know what we were doing. Again, a carefully considered compromise emerged as the process unfolded. To get CEPA off the ground, we decided to plan all of the sessions in advance. But during the meetings, we have tried—largely unsuccessfully—to encourage residents to take over and lead the discussions.

Likewise, we struggled over revealing the full plan of the sessions. Some of us thought that presenting a completed plan would discourage people from realizing they could redirect the sessions; others thought that failing to tell them what was planned would be even more manipulative. So, as the process moved forward, we decided to share plans for the upcoming session and ask the residents for their suggestions and assent. Few changes were made. During periods of critical self-reflection at the end of each session, feedback from residents has generally indicated that they are comfortable with the direction of the discussions. But they have also expressed concerns, on more than one occasion, that they do not understand the relevance of some points and want to move more quickly into planning activities.

Two further examples. In planning the sessions, we decided to devote one meeting to a discussion of the historical relationship between Puerto Rico and the United States. Here, the tensions between a critical empowerment model and a participatory model became most apparent. On the one hand, some of us thought it was important to make clear the connection between the history of the United States' imperialist domination and the disproportionate share of health burdens now borne by the Puerto Rican peoples. On the other hand, other members wanted to hear personal migration stories, see where the discussion led, and work with any insights people might share about their experience. So we were again faced with questions about how to proceed.

In the first round of discussions, we tried to prepare a concise history of Puerto Rico's colonial status. It was, of course, impossible to cover a complete history in such a short period of time. One coalition member ended up presenting a long lecture that took up almost the entire time that evening. The community voices were left out, the residents reduced to a passive role of being fed information. The session jarred us into thinking about the seductiveness of power and control, of prescribing a correct way of thinking, and the challenges of engaging in truly mutual dialogue and deliberation.

Similarly, we felt obligated to present a clinical perspective on HIV transmission. We invited a guest speaker to another session, trying to prepare her for the participatory educational process. Despite the best laid plans, the guest speaker wound up dominating the session and the residents were again treated as empty vessels waiting to be filled.

As was the case after each session, we took time afterwards to discuss these sessions and reflect self-critically on the experience, coming face to face with the possibilities and limits of creating an open public space. The experience brought home how difficult it is to set up a process that fosters autonomy, solidarity, and mutual respect and how difficult it is not to assume a controlling role in telling people what (we think) they need to know.

The coalition members and staff shared their concerns with the residents at the next meeting. Collectively, we decided to repeat the AIDS 101 session, this time, however, listening to what each of us already knew about HIV. The candor of admitting our mistakes, dropping any pretensions as experts with answers about how people should live their lives, changed the tone and dynamic of the meetings. The distance between program developers and program recipients narrowed. Community residents, coalition members, and staff came a little closer as they saw that answers to questions about how to live in the face of the threat of AIDS cannot be dictated.

Looking back on the struggles and occasional false steps, we have been impressed by the benefits of this project. The most moving experience has been a rekindling of pride in Puerto Rican identity. The sense of confusion and ambivalence about having a "dual identity" has been discussed openly for the first time for many. Discussions about the influence of cultural roles and how they shape perceptions, both positively and negatively, have been frank, personal, and collectively liberating. The experience has reconnected each of us with the bonds of community.

9

JUSTICE, CARING, RESPONSIBILITY

This final chapter turns to a discussion of values that matter. Up to this point, no attempt has been made to specify any such values. The preceding pages have put forward the idea that human well-being is characterized by living a life of integrity, as individuals and as a society. We flourish as human beings through living lives in accordance with values of human significance, but there is no one single conception of the good life. The values that people consider significant are plural and not necessarily harmonious nor compatible with one another. The tragedy of the human condition flows from the fact that often we must choose between conflicting goods and values that irreconcilably tug on our conscience. In these situations, we must use judgment, making qualitative discriminations of worth, with insight and sensitivity to the specific context and our clearest, most refined interpretation of the good to be achieved and the values that bear on the situation. We must exercise the faculty of practical reason to make the best decision in light of the particular circumstances.

While plural in number, the kinds of values that matter are not infinite. In the press of instrumental reason and ethical skepticism fostered by modern science, we have developed a kind of self-willed inarticulacy about the good.[1] Yet various scholars have tried in recent years to identify a number of universal values.[2] To begin a discussion of values that matter and conclude this text, I discuss three values that are essential for human well-being. Acting on recommendations in the last chapter about the kinds of research the field needs most, I will try to clarify certain aspects regarding their interpretation. Three values indispensable for achieving human well-being are justice, caring, and responsibility.

JUSTICE

The concept of justice has been central to human understandings of socially significant values since the dawn of recorded history. Justice has long been understood to be the bridge linking integrity and happiness. It offends one's sense of justice when people who lead good lives suffer. Classical philosophers thought that living a life of moral integrity was sufficient to produce happiness, but we now know that this is not always so. Bad things happen to good people. We no longer believe that righteous living guarantees happiness, nor that people flourish only through living life attuned to values that matter. Good people suffer and the wicked sometimes prosper, as John Kekes notes, "even in the long run, even when all things are considered."[3] Thus, we have an interest in promoting justice because we want to bring goodness and happiness more closely together. Moreover, because no amount of individual effort could possibly overcome many of life's misfortunes, we recognize that the prospects for individual well-being depend on the justice of social conditions. The topic of justice frequently crops up in public health meetings. The political scientist Dan Beauchamp has even equated public health with social justice.[4] Yet there are ambiguities in popular use of the term. Two issues in particular—the conflict between universal and communitarian concepts of justice and the contradictory uses of the word justice—have given rise to considerable confusion.

In the modern era, the same Enlightenment dream that led to the triumph of scientific reasoning inspired the hope that one universal, eternally true system of ethics could be established. But perceptions of the irrationality of human values (perceptions derived from the inability to have found a neutral procedure to verify their validity) has led the modern world to give priority to the right over the good and to try to develop an ethical and political system that would remain neutral with respect to the latter. By focusing on questions about what is right, we keep alive the Enlightenment dream of discovering a universal set of rules that would enable us to resolve clashes regarding differing conceptions of the good life for human beings. The two most prominent contemporary spokepersons for this universal rule-procedural ethic are John Rawls and Jurgen Habermas.[5] As we shall see in a moment, misunderstandings arise when the universalist approach runs into conflict with communitarian conceptions of justice based on local, culture-bound conceptions of the good.

The second source of confusion follows from the fact that the same word, "justice," is used to refer to two different understandings of the good life for human beings.[6] One understanding of justice is based on the concept of desert—rewarding people proportionately for their contributions to the common good. A second interpretation is based on equality—seeing human beings as inherently morally equal, and therefore seeing large disparities in the distribution of material wealth as morally reprehensible. Hence, a second source of misunderstanding arises because two different underlying conceptions of the good are being envisioned when people claim their actions are being taken to promote the cause of justice, one based on merit and the other on equality.

On the first point, the best known and most outstanding contemporary attempt to establish a universal set of rule procedures for resolving moral conflicts is John Rawls's *A Theory of Justice*. In this paragon of modern thought, Rawls identifies two rules of justice that he argues will enable humankind to resolve disputes fairly and justly: "First: each person is to have an equal right to the most extensive liberty compatible with a similar liberty for others. Second: social and economic inequalities are to be arranged such that they are both (a) reasonably expected to be to everyone's advantage, and (b) attached to positions and offices open to all."[7]

Critics of Rawls point out two major problems with his theory.[8] MacIntyre and Taylor provide numerous examples of situations where these rules do not provide sufficient guidance for resolving common real-world moral conflicts, e.g., debates about abortion, welfare, taxation, affirmative action, and the rights of indigenous peoples.[9] When faced with real moral dilemmas, Rawls's procedures fail to establish a clear hierarchical rank ordering that stipulates which claim takes precedence.[10] Hence, Rawls's theory fails to accomplish its own stated aims. Second, many philosophers have identified problems with the "original position" invoked by Rawls (i.e., Rawls derives his two rules of justice by asking what principles people would come up with if they were, hypothetically, to meet behind a "veil of ignorance" in a situation where they did not know their own material circumstances). The problem is that the original position is, in effect, Rawls's backdoor way of smuggling in his conception of the good. His theory is tacitly premised on the value of individual equality. As Nagel makes clear, "The original position seems to presuppose not just a neutral theory of the good, but a liberal individualistic one."[11]

In combination, the problem with Rawls's theory of justice is that it tries to establish value-neutral rules for adjudicating value conflicts when, in effect, these rules presuppose and produce a liberal egalitarian understanding of the good life for human beings. Even so, his two rules do not work. They are too abstract to provide much help in resolving actual disputes. This flaw becomes apparent when the goods at stake are difficult to compare with one another; it is impossible in these situations to decide what it means to arrange inequalities to everyone's advantage. What institutional arrangements are we supposed to make to reduce inequalities when one group has an interest in securing certain goods (e.g., a woman's right to choose) and another group other, different, incommensurable types of goods (e.g., the protection of fetal life)? The first source of confusion comes about as a consequence of thinking that we have, or are soon going to find, one universal rule-procedural ethical system. Critics point out that we have not found one yet, and it is probably not in the cards.

The second criticism is that Rawls's theory presumes one particular vision of the human good. While Rawls may claim to have discovered a neutral procedure for adjudicating claims, he has in fact implicitly based his theory of justice on one partial, yet undeniably outstanding, understanding of the good. In his view, justice is concerned with promoting human equality. But his definition of justice conflicts with another well-known interpretation, that of desert.

In contrast to Rawls's liberal egalitarian view of justice, John Kekes presents the concept of justice based on desert.[12] In classical philosophical thought, according to Kekes, both moral worth and human satisfaction were seen to derive from the same source, namely, the extent to which one's life approximated an ideal of the good. But unlike Socrates, we now recognize that this ancient ideal is mistaken, that integrity and happiness may diverge. But even though we know that integrity is not sufficient for flourishing, we continue to believe that it *ought* to be. The call of justice beckons us to try to do the best we can to close the gap, to make being good and being happy coincide as much as possible. As a society, we believe that good actions should lead to happiness, evil deeds to misery, and that happiness or misery ought to be commensurate with the goodness or malevolence of people's conduct.[13] Taylor calls this the "contribution principle," differences in contributions justify differences in remuneration.[14] The idea that people ought to get what they deserve is at the core of this understanding of the meaning of justice. For justice's sake, we try to organize our social institutions such that the likelihood of realizing happiness is high when people live with integrity. The extent to which living a life of integrity leads to happiness is a measure of the extent to which justice prevails.

Taylor expands on the idea of justice based on desert:

> The basic intuition underlying justice is this: in any common attempt to achieve the good, all genuine collaborators benefit from the contributions of the others. They are in a sense all in each other's debt. But since some will make a more signal contribution, the mutual debt may not be entirely reciprocal . . . it is clear that more is owed to these outstanding contributors. They merit more than the rest. . . . This intuition of rightful distribution by desert among associates seems very deeply embedded in human consciousness. . . . Let's say that there are medals to be handed out for valour, or distinguished service. Does anyone doubt that our two outstanding figures above merit them? That it would be a rank injustice to give them to others instead, who had done nothing outstanding?[15]

In this reading, justice involves the allocation of desert. As Kekes says, wisdom is essential for knowing what is good and justice is the value we place on arranging social conditions to support living according to that conception. Promoting justice involves putting our institutions in order, organizing them so that they allocate benefits to promote living in accordance with society's understanding of the good life for human beings. The justice of social conditions is assessed by the extent to which a society's social institutions give credit to those who contribute to human welfare, penalize those who detract from it, and render restitution proportional to the respective acts. To advance the cause of justice, we try to reform institutions along lines that make them ever more closely approximate the ideal of extending rewards and retributions commensurate with the quality of lives. Conscientious acts deserve praise; work deserves wages; kindness, gratitude; criminal acts, imprisonment; and so on.

An important point here is that different societies have different conceptions of the good, and hence reward different kinds of contributions accordingly. Some see the good in individual liberty, others put greater weight on familial and communal obligation. In contrast with universalist conceptions of justice, the idea that different societies might hold different values and assign different weights to various kinds of contributions introduces a communitarian understanding of justice. In terms of communitarian ideals, the pursuit of justice is inextricably tied to promoting local, culture-bound beliefs about what constitutes a valuable contribution to the common good.[16]

Now we can see another common source of confusion concerning the types of actions invoked in the name of justice. Viewed from a slightly different angle, both Rawls and Kekes are arguing for a concept of justice based on desert, although Rawls's commitments are obscured by his claims of value neutrality. Once the assumptions inherent in Rawls's original position are made evident, we can see that he is asserting that all human beings—as individuals, as individual bearers of human dignity—deserve and should be treated with equal respect. Whatever else they might do, we should categorically respect each person because they are members of the human race. The modern world deeply cherishes the sovereignty of the individual. Proponents of a liberal political position thus advocate that people *deserve* an equality of condition because they are human beings whose dignity must be supported and preserved. In contrast, conservatives advocate a meritocracy: people deserve to be rewarded proportionately, commensurate with what they contribute to society. (We can see how this position fits neatly with a capitalist economy and a market system for distributing goods.) At bottom, conflicts over what it means to have a just society in large part derive from underlying conflicts in conceptualizing the good life for human beings. "Each side is pointing to a *different* good," Taylor notes. "They may indeed be rivals, and in that sense incompatible; but they are still both *goods*."[17] One side envisions equality in advocating justice, the other side due compensation for meritorious contributions. It is confusing—and people often talk right past one another—when two very different ideas of where we are headed as a society are invoked in the same name of justice. Once we see more clearly the crux of the debate, then possibilities for moving beyond seemingly intractable impasses could open up.

One possibility for resolving these competing understandings of the requirements of justice might reside in the Aristotelian principle of "proportionate equality."[18] As should be clear by now, Aristotle believed this condition cannot be determined through establishing a priori rules for distributing goods, but rather must be achieved through vigorous moral and political debate about how we can best balance these competing conceptions of the just social conditions in light of present circumstances. Often, it is the failure to see the legitimacy of these competing convictions (i.e., the conflicting demands of justice) that muddies discussions of policy issues germane to health and well-being. These tensions are apparent in four topical issues critical to health promotion. In the future of health promotion, I believe that promoting discussion, debate, and action on these issues in civil society will be essential to achieve a greater measure of individual and community well-being. Community residents may be mobilized around more immediate concerns, such as infant mortality, substance abuse, or AIDS, but it is shortsighted to think we can devise technical solutions to these problems without addressing questions about the justice of social conditions.

The first issue is poverty. Liberals argue that poverty is degrading to the human condition, that it makes a mockery of human autonomy, denigrates the moral equality of individuals, and breeds severe social pathologies. Among conservatives, the justification for its perpetuation is that people are poor because they are not willing to work or that public support fosters dependency.[19] Poor people are only getting what they deserve.[20]

Several thoughts for consideration. First, no matter how hard people try, the economy is not now set up to allow everyone to work. Many people cannot find work through no fault of their own. When the stock market reacts or the Federal Reserve enacts policies to fight inflation that counteract gains in employment, they create obstacles no individual can overcome. Even with the economy booming, millions of Americans remain unemployed. Justice calls us to reform these institutions to better approximate the ideal of desert for one's contributions. Everyone who wants to work should be able to find decent work. A 4-day work week would open up many employment opportunities. Second, the conservative position, founded on a radically atomized view of individual merit, needs to be challenged. It fails to acknowledge the countless ways in which individuals get ahead because of preexisting social privilege, more often than not, to an extent on par with any outcomes that are the result of their own individual initiative. Myths of Horatio Alger are thrown up in a far too one-sided, unrealistic, and obsessive manner.[21] Third, all of us need to recognize that there are competing goods, both legitimate, at stake here. As a society, we may want to strive for more proportionate equality, to borrow Aristotle's understanding of the just society, bringing these competing goods (desert and equality) into greater equilibrium. Even conservative pundits lament the fact that American society now has the greatest inequities in the distribution of wealth in the world.[22] We need to narrow the gap between the rich and the poor if we ever want to achieve any kind of social well-being.

As a first priority, we must work to eliminate poverty among children. Children do not deserve to grow up destitute. They have done nothing that could possibly justify the hardships that poverty visits upon them. In Holyoke, 71.4% of Latino children under 12 are growing up in poverty. If the field is serious about protecting and promoting their health, then the justice of social conditions must be at the forefront of our educational efforts and public discussions. In a society as wealthy as ours, the continued tolerance of children living in poverty is unconscionable. School-based drug prevention programs are not enough. The field of health promotion needs to promote sustained substantive public discussions about the ways we might better organize social and economic institutions, locally and nationally, to bring children's prospects for happiness more in line with their moral desert. There is precedent. Mindful of the value we attach to justice, the nation has largely eliminated poverty among the elderly. The success of Social Security should encourage us all to see that we can expand the sphere of just social conditions.

The second issue is racial discrimination. The need to promote public discussion and to come to a better understanding of the relationship between race and justice cannot be overstated. Because of the way race is the subtext in discussions of poverty,[23] there may be nothing now more injurious to our social well-being than racial antagonisms. In Holyoke, the school system and the health department are funded by local property taxes; race is a major factor in determining levels of support. But it is a difficult question to sort out how to proceed from where we are now toward a more just society. The underlying concepts of equality and desert have become deeply entangled in discussions about race relations.

Cornel West has written eloquently and disturbingly about the prevalence of nihilism and despair in the African-American community.[24] Affirmative action was an attempt to redress historical wrongs; the recent retreat from this program cannot be reassuring to people of color that personal integrity will be enough to ensure that they can find a job, afford decent housing, and make ends meet. The downside of desert, allocating rewards on the basis of competitive success, is that it constantly verges on collapse into images of social inferiority. When people lose their conviction that living honorably, by itself, will be duly rewarded by society, they may sink into a state of not caring about the consequences of their actions. They become unmindful, seeking solace through whatever means offer opportunity. Crime, violence, teen pregnancy, and drug abuse are products of despair. We are never going to make progress on these issues until we sort out the relationship between equality and desert with respect to race and justice in our society.

Many people feel that punishing such behaviors is giving people what they deserve. But as unemployment rates make plain, social problems cannot be reduced to the sum of individual failings. The call of justice beckons us to fulfill our collective responsibility to transform social institutions to promote the common good and create a society in which we can all live together decently. Health educators can promote these discussions in Holyoke and in cities and neighborhoods across the nation.

The third area of concern is access to health care. Here we need to challenge the idea that the market offers a model of just social relations. The idea that we would consciously set out to create a society in which only people who can afford to pay are entitled to medical care and 43 million people are denied access debases the concept of justice. On the contrary, Beauchamp argues that a renewed push for universal access to medical care offers a prime opportunity for rekindling public discussions and debate about the common good.[25] Like education, environmental safeguards, and police, fire, and military protections, the provision of many social goods honors our collective interdependency. Beauchamp makes a strong plea to move beyond narrow instrumental, cost–benefit analyses about whether universal access will improve overall the health status of the population (while reducing costs) and to shift the terms of the debate to recognize that the provision of certain social goods, such as health care, serves to define the kind of people and kind of nation we aspire to be: "My point is this: Health care reform is about strengthening the body politic, strengthening the ways in which we are a people and a community."[26] Everyone deserves access to medical care because the preservation of human dignity demands the alleviation of unnecessary suffering.

The fourth area to address is the relationship between justice and health. Many of us harbor shades of the belief that one's health is some sort of manifestation of cosmic justice. If people do not live right, they get what they deserve: disease, pain, suffering, disability, or premature death. Nowhere is this fallacious thinking more glaring than in insinuations that gay people deserve AIDS. Human immunodeficiency virus is an infectious agent, not divine retribution.

These views derive from the collapse of the idea of living well into physical fitness. Health is not the same as well-being and regimens of diet and exercise are not the same as living with integrity. Many people bemoan a creeping moralistic undertone in health promotion. The charges are warranted to the extent that we have allowed the ends of achieving human well-being to become narrowed and constricted to attaining the objectives of physical fitness. Then, befuddled by claims of an objective "value-neutral" science, we fool ourselves into thinking that health promotion has nothing to do with telling people how we think they ought to live. Let me be clear: the purpose of this book is to claim that health promotion is inescapably—and commendably—a moral and political endeavor. We need to think and to talk more about how people should live, especially as a society with collective responsibilities. But the field also needs to recognize that prescriptions of the good life are open for discussion, that biological viability is not the highest human goal, and that efforts to exercise the power of behavioral control are sadly misguided. The field comes off sounding moralistic when it thinks it knows how people should live and confuses having a strong body with living a good life. Smoking or being overweight tells us little about people's character, except perhaps that the pursuit of physical fitness is not among their most important goals.

Victim-blaming is an outgrowth of the collapse of well-being into physical fitness. As the field avidly proclaims the behavioral determinants of health, many have come to believe that, if someone has a heart attack, he is only getting what he deserves. People are increasingly being blamed for their illnesses, in no small measure because the field has been so successful in fingerpointing "bad" choices.[27] As we move forward, we must not lose sight of the fact that people still get sick through no fault of their own.

Finally, there are other issues, besides smoking and weight control, which may be more important in promoting human well-being. To be sure, the field has a responsibility to inform people about the causes of biological breakdowns. But from there, our principal priority must be in supporting people to improve their own capacity for practical autonomy. Instead of behavior modification, it is time to start helping people become more mindful about their choices, become clearer about the value of a particular course of action, become more discerning and insightful about whether their initial inclinations might have been roused by misdirected motives, and become more conscious of collective responsibilities to create a just society.

Justice is one value that matters. It is essential for realizing human well-being. As Kekes writes, justice is the difference between a barbaric existence in which we get what we deserve only by chance and civilized existence in which human happiness is ever more progressively joined to human integrity.[28] Individual well-being depends mightily on the justice of social conditions. Often, Kekes notes, the cause of justice must start with the relief of injustices. Poverty, racial discrimination, the lack of access to medical care, and the propensity to blame people for getting sick are four areas in which the field of health promotion can start work to alleviate current injustices.

CARING AND RESPECT

Caring is the expression of solidarity with fellow community members. It is bearing witness for their welfare. It is embodied in social practices that strengthen people's dignity and autonomy. But the value of caring is being drained these days. As caring has increasingly come to be equated with curing, many health care providers, especially in the nursing profession, see signs that technological procedures for effecting cures are displacing the moral dimensions of caring practices. These moral dimensions are centered on respect for the individual and the affirmation of human dignity.

In reflecting on the social practice of caring in the helping professions, Bellah makes an important distinction:

> The distinction needs to be drawn between caring as a sentimental psychological attitude and caring as responsible practice, aware of its own limits. . . . Genuine caring is a practice based on moral commitments, with which certain subjective feelings may or may not be associated, but it is not primarily a psychological orientation. Genuine caring does not see those in need primarily as victims. Genuine caring involves a profound sense of moral responsibility, but it does not imagine that caregivers have the technology or the power to heal all wounds and cure all ills.[29]

Jean Bethke Elshtain elaborates:

> [Pope] John Paul's name for this alternative aspiration is "solidarity," not "a feeling of vague compassion or shallow distress at the misfortunes of so many people" but a determination "to commit oneself to the common good; that is to say, to the good of all and of each individual because we are really responsible for all." Through solidarity, John Paul said, we *see*, "the 'other' . . . not just as some kind of instrument . . . but as our 'neighbor,' a 'helper' . . . to be made a sharer on par with ourselves in the banquet of life to which we are all equally invited by God."[30]

Caring is the social practice of accepting responsibility for the well-being of fellow community members. But the deeper dimensions of caring are being depleted, in a two-step process. First, the larger meaning is being supplanted by a narrower, instrumental view of care giving as administering treatments. As the power of science has grown, to care for people has increasingly come to mean nothing more, or less, than to cure them.[31] Granted, effecting cures is a powerful expression of caring. But that power does not capture the full dimensions of its meaning or significance. Nor does it help us to understand what it means to care for others outside of the use of high-tech treatment. When giving care is reduced to administering therapeutic technologies, the moral dimensions of caring practices are forfeit, a loss that becomes painfully apparent at the limits of technology when there are no more cures to dispense.

In the second step of depletion, without such deeper understandings to draw on, subjective feelings of pity or sympathy are all that remain in caring for others. The emotional reserves of the caregiver are then left to assume a burden far greater than they can bear. That common modern professional affliction, "burnout," is often the result of viewing caring as nothing more than personal kindness or empathy in lieu of effective treatment.

In surveying the state of the nursing profession, Susan Phillips laments the erosion in understanding:

> Increasingly in the helping professions, personhood and caring have been eclipsed by the depersonalizing procedures of . . . technological problem-solving and the techniques and relations of the marketplace. . . . The objectification of persons within the rela-

tionship of caregiving leaves many caregivers frustrated, confused, and ashamed of their genuinely compelled caring while many receivers of care are humiliated, angry, and alienated. Our culture has omitted a significant dimension of human being from consideration and attention. Iris Murdoch writes, "The charm and power of technology and the authority of the 'scientific outlook' conceal the speed with which the idea of the responsible moral spiritual individual is being diminished."[32]

Phillips identifies two goods lost in the transformation of caring into curing. The first is respect: the loss of attention to the individual as a unique person with his or her own singular personality and projects. The second is responsibility: the loss of appreciation for the types of social practices that cultivate responsible selfhood. As caring has increasingly come to rely on the power of science, the helping professions have increasingly become caught up in social practices that diminish respect for the individual and deny people responsibility for their actions.

The value of scientific research is directly proportional to the generalizability of its findings. Scientific theory is useless without generalizations beyond the particular observation on which it is based; it is the very breadth of its application that gives scientific theory its power and utility.[33] The whole of health promotion research is currently directed toward identifying such generalizable risk factors. When National Institute on Drug Abuse (NIDA) states that it is soliciting research proposals to develop strategies that are "universally effective" to prevent drug use, it is not looking for nor interested in developing strategies tailored to the individual. When practitioners fail to follow drug prevention curriculum instructions precisely, they are accused of undermining or attenuating its effectiveness. It is in this sense that Phillips perceives that scientific reasoning is depersonalizing. In searching for generalizations, the scientific outlook looks in quite the opposite direction from a caring orientation based on respect for the individual.

"Respect for persons," Steven Lukes writes, "requires, among other things, that we regard and act toward individuals in their concrete specificity, that we take full account of their specific aims and purposes and of their own definitions of their (social) situations."[34] Caring requires treating people with respect. Out of respect for the difficulty of the task of giving meaning to life that all of us must face, we honor the effort by paying attention to the distinguishing details of a person's life. We suspend ready labels and stereotypes, wanting instead to know individuals in their complexity. The more we genuinely care about a person, the more we want to appreciate what makes him or her unique.

To say that we respect someone also means that we conscientiously avoid violating or interfering with that person's particular wishes and intentions. When we act as if we know better what other people want or need, we denigrate that respect. It is a direct assault on individual integrity. When we presume that our goals are more important than their goals, we deny them their dignity. "A person is free in so far as his actions are his own," Lukes writes, "that is in so far as they result from decisions and choices which he makes as a free agent, rather than as the instrument or object of another's will or as a result of external or internal forces independent of his will. His autonomy consists precisely in this self-determined deciding and choosing. That autonomy is reduced in so far as his actions are determined elsewhere than by his conscious 'self.'"[35] Kant forcefully stated the relevant moral principle: "Act so that you treat humanity, whether in your own person or that of another, always as an end and never as a means only." Selznick hammers in the point: "The claims of efficiency are strong, but they cannot justify practices that reduce human beings to 'means only.' Such practices make them victims of domination."[36]

In searching for the causes of human behavior, the commitment to the scientific method is antithetical to the idea that people are capable of making autonomous responsible choices. The presumption that behavior is determined by antecedent risk factors stands in direct contradiction to the idea that people have the ability to make free choices for which they may be held accountable. By perpetuating a social practice premised on discovering what causes a person to behave a certain way, the field of health promotion undercuts the idea of moral responsibility. Health promotion researchers assume that there are independent forces that make people do what they do, and, through the power of science, they plan to rid them of those errant antecedent social and psychological risk factors.

But when people are thought not to be responsible for their behavior, the field loses sight of the source of human dignity, that which makes human beings worthy of respect. We think that human beings have a special dignity, that they deserve our respect, because no matter how unfortunate, they still retain the capacity to do what they ought to do, unlike any other creature on earth. When we treat them as if their choices were foreordained, we become blind to that exceptional mark of human existence that gives human beings their dignity. To think that effecting changes in others' behaviors is the best expression of caring for them is, therefore, tragically misguided.

Caring is better expressed in social practices that foster human dignity, autonomy, and integrity by treating people with respect as unique individuals. Caring is standing in solidarity with fellow community members, paying homage to our interdependence. Phillips and Benner make this clear: "Caring relationships set up the possibility of mutual realization, not a power discourse in which one person gives, helps, and does not learn from the other, while the other person merely receives and learns. . . . [On the contrary,] the caregiver learns and is transformed by the caregiving relationship."[37]

RESPONSIBILITY

Throughout this book, I have tried to indicate how the capacity for moral responsibility—for evaluating first-order desires and consciously choosing, for good reason, one course over another in order to become the kind of person we admire and live the kind of life we think most worthwhile—is a unique quality of human existence. I have discussed social practices that undermine this sense of responsibility. I want to conclude with reflections about how we might better nurture the value of taking responsibility for our actions.

The philosopher Herbert Fingarette identifies two elements in the origin of a sense of responsibility: "One is that of acceptance, of commitment, care, and concern, and of attendant elements of choice and the creativity of choice; the other dimension is that of the 'forms of life,' initially socially given and ultimately socially realized, which constitute the form and content of responsibility." He continues, "Responsibility emerges where the individual accepts as a matter of personal concern something which society offers to his concern."[38] Concern for the "forms of life," the social practices of one's community, is indispensable for the emergence of a sense of responsibility. The emotional bond is the impetus for thinking about the effects of different courses of action on others in one's community.

The desire to act responsibly is not something that can be instrumentally induced, not something that can be effected through skilled scientific techniques, however powerful. We cannot compel people to care about, and so feel responsible for, their world. We can only hold up what we think valuable for them to see. People come to assume a sense of responsibility as they become concerned about, as they accept as part of their concerns, the ways of life that a community offers. Responsibility grows with the recognition and approval of one's attachment to the given forms of social life. The genesis of responsible personhood is the perception of value in the walks of life around us.

In contrast, "Meaninglessness (a place of not caring)," write Patricia Benner and Judith Wrubel, "and *anomie* (the loss of a feeling of belonging) are the positions most bereft of coping options, because all things appear equal—nothing stands out as relatively more important or less important or inviting. Nothing really matters."[39] If people cannot see the value, the intrinsic, internal good, in their community's social practices, life appears barren, empty. And if nothing seems worthwhile, there is nothing to build on. The grounds for forming the commitments that give life purpose and meaning never materialize. It is the essence of nihilism, seeing nothing of value.

When we find something we care about, we find our bearings, a direction, a point on the horizon that stands out, a destination worth heading toward.[40] Without these "horizons of value," as Taylor calls them, we have no points of reference, no basis for evaluating any internal impulses, nothing to do but to act on them since there is nothing relative to which we can determine whether they are worthwhile or not.[41] If there is nothing outside ourselves that we care about, nothing given by the existing world, then it does not matter what we are doing or where we are going because all points appear indistinguishable. It matters to us whether our actions might distress others when we care about them and their welfare. It matters whether we choose one course of action over another only if we care about the kind of life one set of practices embodies over another. Otherwise, we become oblivious, irresponsible.

We can begin to see the mutually reinforcing relationships among justice, caring, and responsibility. For individuals to want to act responsibly, to want to evaluate their desires in relation to the larger society in which they live, they must care about that community. People care about their community when social conditions afford them reasonable hope that living responsibly will enable them to live well. Conversely, people feel hopeless when social conditions fall short of how they believe those conditions ought to be, when there appears to be no connection between acting responsibly and gaining happiness. In such times and places, people will not care about the effect of their actions on their community, will not care to act responsibly, because such conduct bears no evident relationship to their well-being, their prospects for living well. Just social conditions are necessary to stave off despair and to promote caring for one's community, creating the emotional bond essential to seeing the value of acting responsibly.

If the seeds of responsibility are planted in the perception of value, then the implications for health promotion are clear. To recall Gadamer's words, "In the end, this is the birth of the concept of reason: the more what is desirable is displayed for all in a way that is convincing to all, the more those involved discover themselves in this common reality."[42] We try to make clear what is good in this life so that others may see its value, and from there, reform, expand and make it better. Community health educators can share what we think is valuable, but we cannot make people feel its grandeur. There are no techniques, no factors to manipulate that will cause them to come to cherish and embrace a way of life. It is a choice they have to make for themselves.

THE PROMISE OF HEALTH PROMOTION

There is an old joke about the number of therapists it takes to change a light bulb. The answer—"Only one, but the light bulb's gotta want to change." The joke is funny, of course, because it points up human folly. The "troubled person's industry," as the sociologist Joe Gusfield aptly refers to our lot,[43] spends too much of its time and energy trying to devise better, more effective light bulb changing techniques when the crux of the matter lies in clarifying what people want.

There are serious problems in our society that the field urgently needs to address. But we need to think more deeply about sources of these problems and reevaluate the means and ends of our response. The field of health promotion needs to reconceptualize the paradigm that frames our thinking about these issues. As professionals, we need to rethink the tools we are using and what they can, and cannot, tell us about the nature of these problems. We need to reevaluate whether methods of research that have proven effective in identifying germs and verifying cause-and-effect relationships are the most well-suited for clarifying values and strengthening judgment. If the source of most contemporary health problems lies in the choices people make about how they want to live their lives, then we need to rethink whether the commitment to an empirical, experimental science is adequate or appropriate for dealing with them.

The predominant value guiding the practice of health promotion today is instrumental efficiency, a value that conflicts with many other socially significant values. The rise of instrumental reason and consequent decline of practical reason have displaced research from studying and clarifying these value conflicts to pursuing the development of more effective techniques. Science cannot tell us which goals are more worthwhile than others, which ways of living more valuable. It cannot tell us how we should live. To pretend that the task of promoting human health is not about trying to figure out how we should live is to lose sight of the ends of achieving health well-being. Human well-being is defined in terms of living with dignity, integrity, autonomy, and responsibility. If the quest for a science of health promotion ever were successful, the very ends that constitute the life most worth living would be destroyed. Physiological functioning could possibly be improved, but it would be at the cost of a life with diminished dignity, integrity, autonomy, and responsibility. The joyless irony here is that this quest is destined for failure.

The meta-narrative of the quest for a science of health promotion is that values cannot ultimately be justified: they are arbitrary and subjective, and therefore people should seek power to make sure they get what they want. The organization and practice of the institution of public health currently reflects these understandings. Public health as an institution is devoted virtually in its entirety to developing more effective techniques to change people's behavior in order to achieve public health goals. In our preoccupation with means, we contribute to the collapse of institutional practices for reflecting upon and clarifying visions of the good life for individuals and communities.

The source of most contemporary health problems lies in the choices people make about how they want to live their lives, and, more fundamentally, in the choices we make as a society about the organization and practices of our social institutions. We need to pay attention to the social practices of our institutions, the goods they seek to promote, and how they nurture the cultivation of certain virtues. Because we care, because we find meaning and value in the profession of service to humankind, and because we have the capacity and the responsibility for choosing the direction we are headed, we have reason to reflect on the practices in which we are engaged and decide the wisest course of action for the future. What is the promise of health promotion? My concern is reflected in current developments in Holyoke.

Gladys is hurrying through the courtyard, on her way to a *charla* ("chat") in an apartment located in one of the scariest, most drug-infested tenement complexes in Holyoke. She knows the family and the neighbors who will be there and is following up on their request for information on AIDS. She has her hands full with a VCR and trips over a syringe discarded in the walkway. This time, she has brought along the state program director, a doctoral candidate at Harvard. Gladys asks her to pick it up, figuring it will be a good trigger for discussion. They see a man overdosed in the hallway, perhaps dying. Residents are hiding behind closed doors, afraid to get involved with the police. Gladys steps over him and calls 911. (Carlos survives; in way of thanks, he develops a *fotonovella* for CEDE.)

Under the auspices of CEDE, Gladys is working to promote prenatal care and reduce infant mortality. Tonight the tenant's apartment has a gaping, drafty hole in the wall and the ceiling leaks. The tenant said last time that he would talk to the landlord, but he is struggling with heroin addiction and so fears he cannot stir things up too much. Gladys is furious. Everything is so hopeless, and all that people are doing is complaining about leaks in the ceiling. She presses the point, "What do you think is going on? What can we do?" She asks them directly about their feelings of hopelessness.

Gladys is ready to start from wherever they want. People are worried about drug dealers. It seems they cannot bring it up directly, so they bring it up indirectly, asking for an educational workshop. The request for a videotape on AIDS is a safe way to get into their larger concerns. She wants them to get organized, but she wants even more for them to figure out their own solutions. Pulling out the discarded needle, the discussion takes off. The tenants have some ideas about what they can do. Some do not have phones, so they devise a system of banging on pipes to alert neighbors to notify the police when they see dealing going on. They are angry about the slow response time of the police. Faced with public pressure, eventually, the police department stations a full-time officer there 24 hours a day. Gladys tells the tenants about building codes and Board of Health regulations, about their right to withhold rent until the building is brought up to the sanitary code. The tenants take the landlord to court and get the building condemned. Gladys refuses to take credit. "You gotta believe in the people," she says.

Often she helps people find a job, going with them to the interviews, helping write letters of application, and appearing in court when necessary. She is negotiating with the local Carpenter's Union now, urging them to set up a training program to impart valuable job skills. What, you may ask, does this have to do with improving compliance with prenatal care and reducing infant mortality? Activists in the field have become quite skilled in making claims about how finding someone a job will eventually lead down the causal chain of events to effect reductions in infant mortality. How else can people like Gladys justify what they do?

There is an alternative. Instead of resorting to these types of rationalizations, I think that programs can be fully responsive to local needs and fully accountable to funding sources, without defining the target population with predetermined behavioral objectives set by state or federal funding agencies. It is eminently feasible for public and private authorities to fund health promotion positions without restricting funding to categorical mandates; they could, instead, provide block grant funding to support local community efforts. Why isn't it enough that, with the support of Gladys and the CEDE program, the residents have cleaned and fixed up the apartments, moved drug dealers out of the apartments, advocated for job training programs, and found people jobs? Programs like Gladys's can be accountable, she can document everything they accomplish, and still let the people themselves decide what they want to do.

Gladys is working with a woman who is pregnant and homeless. The woman is not sure where or how she is going to get her next meal. The idea of "educating" her about keeping prenatal appointments seems a bit shortsighted to Gladys. CEDE came up for refunding in 1996. The renewal grant application requires the enumeration of specific operational objectives. Each year, the state department of public health steps up its demand for numbers—number of client contacts, number of patients enrolled, number of educational presentations, number of appointments kept. The application form now requires specification of the behavioral change theoretical framework the agency plans to use. It requires the itemization of predefined outcome measures. In an era of managed care, the renewal grant calls for the utilization of a case management model.

Fearing community will be replaced with management, Gladys quietly exults when she learns CEDE has not been refunded.

Notes

CHAPTER 1: DISQUIETUDES

1. All articles appeared in New York *Times*, February 14, 1997.

2. The term "health promotion" will be used here to refer to all those planned, intentional activities designed to reduce the incidence and prevalence of those diseases that have primarily a sociobehavioral etiology (as opposed to diseases caused principally by infectious agents, genetic, or environmental factors). A convenient catalogue of the scope of health promotion activities is the list of topics identified under Health Promotion in the United States Surgeon General's *Healthy People 2000*, which is comprised of smoking, alcohol and other drugs, nutrition, physical fitness/exercise, family planning, mental health, and violence. Also, some people make a distinction between "health promotion" and "health education," where health promotion refers to activities targeting broader social, economic, and environmental change and health education is said to focus more narrowly on providing information to individuals. But, following Glanz, Lewis, and Rimer, I will use these terms interchangeably. See Glanz, Lewis, and Rimer, *Health Behavior and Health Education*, 1997, pp. 6–7.

3. Let me reiterate that many diseases, such as many cancers, are *not* caused by behaviors or lifestyles, but are due, for example, to toxic environmental exposures or genetic predisposition. There are other public health problems, such as hunger and homelessness, over which individuals exercise little control. I do not want to suggest that individuals are to blame for becoming ill with these types of diseases nor are they the subject of this book. See Note 1 above.

4. Callahan, "Health and Society: Some Ethical Imperatives," 1977.

5. See, for example, Nyswander, "The Open Society: Its Implications for Health Educators," 1967; Beauchamp, "Public Health as Social Justice," 1976; Brown and Margo, "Health Education: Can the Reformers be Reformed?" 1978; Freudenberg, "Training Health Educators for Social Change," 1984; Labonte, "Social Inequality and Healthy Public Policy," 1986; and Minkler, "Health Education, Health Promotion, and the Open Society: An Historical Perspective," 1989.

6. Lofquist, *The Technology of Prevention Workbook*, 1989.

7. Gitlan, *The Twilight of Common Dreams*, 1995, p. 200.

8. Anderson notes, "Most social scientists are epistemologically quite uncurious and, as a consequence, many verge on dogmatism and some, in fact, achieve it." Anderson, *Prescribing the Life of the Mind*, 1993, p. 135.

9. Bok, *State of the Nation*, 1996, p. 1.

10. Miringoff, *1996 Index of Social Health*, 1996.

11. Miringoff, *1996 Index of Social Health*, 1996, p. 7.

12. Bennett, *The Index of Leading Cultural Indicators*, 1994, p. 8.

13. Bronfenbrenner, et al., *The State of Americans*, 1996, p. 260.

14. Sandel, *Democracy's Discontent*, 1996, p. 3.

15. Huba, et al., "Framework for an Interactive Theory of Drug Use," 1980.

16. For summary reviews, see Susser, "The Tribulations of Trials—Intervention in Communities," 1995; and, Pancer and Nelson. "Community-Based Approaches to Health Promotion: Guidelines for Community Mobilization," 1990.

17. Maccoby, et al., "Reducing the Risk of Cardiovascular Disease: Effects of a Community-Based Campaign on Knowledge and Behavior," 1977; Stanford Five City Project Research Group, "The Stanford Five City Project: Design and Methods," 1985.

18. Carlaw, et al., "Organization for a Community Cardiovascular Health Program: Experiences from the Minnesota Heart Health Program," 1984; Minnesota Heart Health Program Research Group, "Community-Wide Prevention of Cardiovascular Disease: Education Strategies of the Minnesota Heart Health Program." *Preventive Medicine*, 15(1):1–17, 1986.

19. Lefebvre, et al., "Theory and Delivery of Health Programming in the Community: The Pawtucket Heart Health Program," 1987; Lefebvre, et al., "Community Intervention to Lower Blood Cholesterol: The 'Know Your Cholesterol' Campaign in Pawtucket, Rhode Island," 1986.

20. Puska, "Community-Based Prevention of Cardiovascular Disease: The North Karelia Project," 1984; North Karelia Project Team, "The Community-Based Strategy to Prevent Coronary Heart Disease: Conclusions from the Ten Years of the North Karelia Project," 1985.

21. Multiple Risk Factor Intervention Trial Research Group (MRFIT), "Multiple Risk Factor Intervention Trial: Risk Factor Changes and Mortality Results," 1982; Multiple Risk Factor Intervention Trial Research Group (MRFIT), "Mortality Rates After 10.5 Years for Participants in the Multiple Risk Factor Intervention Group," 1990.

22. COMMIT Research Group, "Community Intervention Trial for Smoking Cessation (COMMIT): I. Cohort Results from a Four-Year Community Intervention," 1995; COMMIT Research Group, "Community Intervention Trial for Smoking Cessation (COMMIT): II. Changes in Adult Smoking Prevalence," 1995.

23. Glanz, Lewis, and Rimer, *Health Behavior and Health Education*, 1997, p. 13.

24. US Department of Health and Human Services, *Alcohol and Health*, 1990.

25. Gerstein and Harwood, *Treating Drug Problems*, 1990.

26. Centers for Disease Control, "Effectiveness of Smoking Control Strategies—United States," 1992.

27. Klem, et al. "A Descriptive Study of Individuals Successful at Long-Term Maintenance of Substantial Weight Loss." 1997.

28. Shilts, *And the Band Played On*, 1987; Green, J., "Just Say No? Flirting with Suicide," 1996.

29. Taylor, *The Malaise of Modernity*, 1992, pp. 1–5.

30. Taylor, *The Malaise of Modernity*, 1992, pp. 1–5.

31. Weber, "The Social Psychology of the World Religions," in Gerth and Mills, *From Max Weber*, 1946, p. 293.

32. Selznick, *The Moral Commonwealth*, 1992, p. 56.

33. See Weber, *The Protestant Ethic and the Spirit of Capitalism*, 1905/1930; Brubaker, *The Limits of Rationality*, 1984, p. 1; Morrison, *Marx, Durkheim, Weber*, 1995, p. 4.

34. Weber, *The Protestant Ethic and the Spirit of Capitalism*, 1958, p. 26; cited in Brubaker, *The Limits of Rationality*, 1984, p. 8, 24.

35. On ideal types, see Weber, *The Methodology of the Social Sciences*, 1949; see also, Buchanan, "An Uneasy Alliance: Combining Qualitative and Quantitative Research Methods," 1992, for an explanation and examples of the use of ideal types in health promotion

research. The idea that there are different kinds of knowledge may initially sound strange. Gardner's *Frames of Mind* (1983), where he discusses multiple kinds of intelligences, and C. P. Snow's famous "two cultures" debate are helpful in thinking about the distinct mindsets.

36. Brubaker, *The Limits of Rationality*, 1984, p. 2.

37. Brubaker, *The Limits of Rationality*, 1984, p. 3; as he continues: "The extension of scientific knowledge, to be sure, enhances man's rational control over social and natural processes. But while this control has made possible dramatic improvements in material well-being, it has also made possible the development of increasingly sophisticated techniques for the 'political, social, educational, and propagandistic manipulation and domination of human beings.' . . . Above all, it is this purely formal character, this indifference to all substantive ends and values, that defines what is unique—as well as what is morally and politically problematic—about Western rationalism." Brubaker, *The Limits of Rationality*, 1984, pp. 3–4, 10, citing Weber in *The Methodology of the Social Sciences*; see also Turner, *Max Weber*, 1992, pp. 11, 115.

38. Larmore, *The Morals of Modernity*, 1996, p. 190.

39. Selznick summarizes the differences in these terms: "Nevertheless, a fundamental tension exists between instrumental rationality and moral [practical] reason. The former depends on definite purposes and clear criteria of cost and achievement, with a natural preference for specialization and for the autonomy of professional or craft decisions. This way of thinking tends to narrow perspectives and limit responsibilities. . . . Moral [practical] reason, by contrast, makes goals problematic and broadens responsibility. It asks: Are the postulated ends worth pursuing, in light of the means they seem to require? Are the institution's values, as presently formulated, worthy of realization? What costs are imposed on *other* ends and *other* values?" Selznick, *The Moral Commonwealth*, 1992, p. 321; see also Kenney, *Aristotle on the Perfect Life*, 1992, p. 1, and Ch. 5.

40. See, for example, Anderson, *Prescribing the Life of the Mind*, 1993; Ingram, *Reason, History, & Politics*, 1995.

41. Larmore, for example, notes, "[Positivism] necessarily regards our moral judgments as expressions of preference and not as potentially a form of knowledge." Larmore, *The Morals of Modernity*, 1996, p. 7.

42. Taylor, "Explanation and Practical Reasoning," 1995, p. 34.

43. Taylor, "Justice After Virtue," 1985, p. 41.

44. Anderson, *Prescribing the Life of the Mind*, 1993, p. 36.

45. Taylor, "Justice After Virtue," 1985, p. 25.

46. The goal of reducing mortality rates is most explicitly evident in the United States Surgeon General's *Promoting Health, Preventing Disease: Objectives for the Nation* (1980); see also Callahan, *False Hopes*, 1998, p. 78, "The priorities of research are equally skewed by placing the struggle against death first on the list (as has been the case for years at the National Institutes of Health)."

47. Selznick, *The Moral Commonwealth*, 1992, p. 321. See note 39 above.

48. See Grossman, "Health for What? Change, Conflict, and the Search for Purpose," 1971; and, Foege, "Public Health and Purpose in Life," 1986, for similar points of view.

49. Glanz, Lewis, and Rimer, *Health Behavior and Health Education*, 1997, p. 25.

50. Glanz, Lewis, and Rimer, *Health Behavior and Health Education*, 1997, p. 26. See also Kipnis, "Accounting for the Use of Behavior Technologies in Social Psychology," 1994, for a significant expansion on this point.

51. Glanz, Lewis, and Rimer, *Health Behavior and Health Education*, 1997, p. 3.

52. Jackson, "Behavioral Science Theory and Principles for Practice in Health Education," 1997, pp. 143–144.

53. Drug Abuse Prevention and Communications Research, Request for Applications # DA-98-006, Release Date: February 20, 1998. National Institute on Drug Abuse of the National Institutes of Health.

54. While a clear succinct statement of the philosophy of logical positivism is difficult to pinpoint, see Carnap, *Testability and Meaning* (1956) and Mill, *Philosophy of Scientific Method* (1950) for highly representative examples. Ingram offers this description: "Following the influential analysis proffered by Karl Popper, Carl Hempel, and Paul Oppenheim, it has been customary to think of causal explanations as *deducing* a description of some particular event E to be explained (the explanandum) from a description of a particular set of conditions C causally related to E, conjoined with an empirical generalization of the form, if C then E (the explanans). . . . As described above, positivism conforms to SR [scientific rationality] in three respects: it defines argumentation (justification) in terms of formal rules of deductive logic, it founds meaning and truth in direct observation, and it equates explanation with determinate causal prediction." Ingram, *History, Reason, and Politics*, 1995, p. 75.

55. On the need to address normative questions that require humanistic and interpretive approaches, see Chs. 3 and 5.

56. See, for example, Winch's *The Idea of a Social Science*, 1958, and Gadamer's *Truth and Method*, 1960.

57. For example, the first article on the "constructivist" paradigm to be published in *Health Education Quarterly* was published in 1996. See Labonte and Robertson, "Health Promotion Research and Practice: The Case for the Constructivist Paradigm," 1996, but to which Glanz, Lewis, and Rimer reply, "It has become increasingly common in the field for work to originate within a constructivist paradigm and then shift toward a focus on answering specific research questions using methodologies from the logical positivist paradigm." Glanz, Lewis, and Rimer, *Health Behavior and Health Education*, 1997, p. 25.

58. For example, influences such as the rise and confluence of a capitalist market economy, a liberal political philosophy, and a utilitarian moral philosophy.

59. Lukes, *Individualism*, 1973, pp. 127–128.

60. Selznick, *The Moral Commonwealth*, 1992, p. 319.

61. Duncan and Cribb, "Helping People Changes—an Ethical Approach?" 1996, p. 340.

62. Taylor, "Justice After Virtue," 1985, p. 31.

63. Bellah, "Social Science as Practical Reason," 1983, p. 35, 43.

CHAPTER 2: CONTEMPORARY THREATS TO HEALTH

1. United States Census Bureau, 1990.

2. All health indicators are courtesy of the Massachusetts Department of Public Health, 1995.

3. Mausner and Bahn, *Epidemiology: An Introductory Text*, 1974, p. 33.

4. The following material is adapted from Chave, "The Origins and Development of Public Health," 1986; Rosen, *A History of Public Health*, 1993; and Buchanan, "The Relevance of Behavioral Research for Public Health Professionals," 1996.

5. Cited in Lilienfeld, *Foundations of Epidemiology*, 1993, pp. 20–21.

6. Rosen, *A History of Public Health*, 1993, pp. 270–319.

7. Rosen, *A History of Public Health*, 1993, pp. 287–290.

8. Terris, "The Epidemiologic Revolution, National Health Insurance, and the Role of Health Departments," 1976.

9. McKeown, *The Role of Medicine: Dream, Mirage, or Nemesis*, 1976.

10. McKinlay and McKinlay, "The Questionable Contribution of Medical Measures to the Decline of Mortality in the United States in the Twentieth Century," 1977.

11. United States Surgeon General, *Healthy People*, 1979, p. 4.

12. United States Surgeon General, *Healthy People*, 1979, p. 7.

13. Dawber, Meadors, and Moore, "Epidemiological Approaches to Heart Disease: The Framingham Study," 1951; Kannel, et al., "Factors of Risk in the Development of Coronary Heart Disease—Six Year Follow-Up Experience: The Framingham Study," 1961.

14. Neubrauer and Pratt, "The Second Public Health Revolution," 1981.

15. Belloc and Breslow, "Relationship of Health Status and Health Practices," 1972.

16. Berkman and Syme, "Social Networks, Host Resistance, and Mortality: A Nine-Year Follow-up Study of Alameda County Residents," 1979.

17. Syme and Berkman, "Social Class, Susceptibility, and Sickness," 1976, p. 1.

18. Marmot, Kogevinas, and Elston, "Social/Economic Status and Disease," 1987.

19. Haan, Kaplan, and Camacho, "Poverty and Health: Prospective Evidence from the Alameda County Study," 1987.

20. Haan, Kaplan, and Camacho, "Poverty and Health: Prospective Evidence from the Alameda County Study," 1987, p. 994.

21. Haan, Kaplan, and Camacho, "Poverty and Health: Prospective Evidence from the Alameda County Study," 1987, p. 994.

22. As a side note, the report received considerable attention because it was the first major official national document to state that medical care makes a relatively minor contribution to the health status of the population as a whole. See LaLonde, *A New Perspective on the Health of Canadians*, 1975.

23. United States Surgeon General, *Healthy People*, 1979, p. 9.

24. Department of Health and Social Security, *Inequalities in Health*, 1980.

25. Greenwald, Cullen, and McKenna, "Cancer Prevention and Control: From Research through Applications," 1987.

26. Cook, et al., "Rules of Evidence and Clinical Recommendations on the Use of Antithrombotic Agents," 1992.

27. Glanz, Lewis, and Rimer, *Health Behavior and Health Education*, 1997, p. 20.

28. Much of the material in this section is revised and adapted from Buchanan and Cernada, "AIDS Prevention Programs: A Critical Review," 1998.

29. See Glanz, Lewis, and Rimer, *Health Behavior and Health Education*, 1997, for a representative list of these theories.

30. Chin and Benne, "General Strategies for Effecting Change in Human Systems," 1985.

31. Among the many possible references describing this planning framework, see Green and Kreuter, *Health Promotion Planning*, 1991.

32. Andersen and Mullner, "Assessing the Health Objectives of the Nation," 1990.

33. Green, "Modifying and Developing Health Behavior," 1984.

34. Green and Kreuter, *Health Promotion Planning*, 1991.

35. Green and Kreuter, *Health Promotion Planning*, 1991: "On the basis of cumulative research on health and social behavior, literally hundreds of factors could be identified that have the potential to influence a given health behavior." p. 28.

36. McLeroy, et al., "An Ecological Perspective on Health Promotion Programs," 1988.

37. All statistics are taken from United States Department of Health and Human Services *Health, United States*, 1994.

38. Anders, *Health Against Wealth*, 1996.

39. Halverson, Kaluzny, and McLaughlin, *Managed Care and Public Health*, 1998.

40. See, for example, Bengen-Seltzer, *Fourth Generation Managed Behavioral Health*, 1997.

41. Nelson, et al., "The State of Research Within Managed Care Plans: 1997 Survey," 1998.

42. Deutsch, "Rewarding Employees for 'Wellness'," 1991.

43. McGinnis and Foege, "Actual Causes of Death in the United States," 1993.

44. Green and Kreuter, *Health Promotion Planning*, 1991, p. 131.

CHAPTER 3: THE LIMITS OF SCIENCE

1. Glanz, Lewis, and Rimer, *Health Education and Health Behavior*, 1997, p. 23.

2. The contemporary conservative British philosopher Michael Oakeshott coined this pair of helpful heuristic labels, respectively, *natural processes* and *social practices*. Natural processes are embedded in the very structure of nature; their occurrence is inherent in the composition and configuration of the constituent elements. Think, for example, of chemical reactions. In contrast, social practices require intelligence. They need to be learned, understood, and granted assent by the performer. Think of any cultural custom, like manners, dress, signs of greeting, etc. Oakeshott, *On Human Conduct*, 1975.

3. For similar positions, see Weed, "Epidemiology, the Humanities, and Public Health," 1995; Lawson and Floyd, "The Future of Epidemiology: A Humanist Response," 1996; Susser and Susser, "Choosing a Future for Epidemiology," 1996; and, Davies, "Health Research: Time for a Methodological Revolution?" 1996.

4. See Buchanan, "An Uneasy Alliance: Combining Qualitative and Quantitative Research Methods," 1992, for a discussion of these different goals, assumptions, and standards.

5. Taylor, "Justice After Virtue," 1985, p. 25.

6. Taylor, "Explanation and Practical Reason," 1995, p. 40.

7. Among many possible accounts of this history, see Tarnas, *The Passion of the Western Mind*, 1991.

8. Berlin, *The Crooked Timber of Humanity*, 1991, p. 5.

9. Taylor, "Explanation and Practical Reason," 1995, p. 46, emphasis in original.

10. Appleby, Hunt, and Jacob, *Telling the Truth about History*, 1994, p. 246.

11. See, for example, Eckert, "Beyond the Statistics of Adolescent Smoking," 1983, in which an anthropological ethnography of adolescent smoking was published in the "Commentary" section of the field's masthead journal.

12. "It has become increasingly common in the field for work to originate within a constructivist paradigm and then shift toward a focus on answering specific research questions using methodologies from the logical positivist paradigm." Glanz, Lewis, and Rimer, *Health Behavior and Health Education*, 1997, p. 25. See also Miles and Huberman, *Qualitative Data Analysis*, 1994, for a similar position placing qualitative methods within the positivist paradigm.

13. Aristotle, *Nichomachean Ethics*, 1962, see Book Six.

14. Nussbaum, *Love's Knowledge*, 1990, pp. 38, 71–72.

15. Nussbaum, *Love's Knowledge*, 1990, p. 39.

16. To anticipate common objections, none of this is to say human action is random and chaotic. It is to say that human behavior gains its regularity and "predictability" not so much because it is caused by inexorable antecedent events, but because we live in a shared world of moral expectations, a world in which people choose, have a right to expect, and partake in shared expectations about how members of that world ought to behave. See Rehg, *Insight and Solidarity*, 1997, p. 25.

17. See Searle, *Minds, Brains, and Science*, 1984; Hollis, *The Philosophy of Social Science*, 1994; and Nagel, *The Last Word*, 1997.

18. Aristotle, *Nichomachean Ethics*, 1962, p. 65.

19. Searle, *Minds, Brains, and Science*, 1984, p. 87.

20. Cited in Selznick, *The Moral Commonwealth*, 1992, p. 44.

21. Credit is usually given to Dilthey for making the original distinction; see Dilthey, *Selected Writings*, 1976. See also Weber, *Economy and Society*, 1978; von Wright, *Explanation and Understanding*, 1971; and Apel, *Understanding and Explanation*, 1984.

22. Brown, Robert, *The Nature of Social Laws*, 1984, p. 15.

23. "Now I have been told by friendly colleagues that this last statement, namely, that human actions are not determined by immutable and universal laws, cannot be proved, and that to assert it is in the nature of metaphysical speculation. Fair enough. You may consider it, then, to be part of my metaphysics that I believe in free will and in choice; that human beings are fundamentally different from orbiting planets and melting ice; and that while we are profoundly influenced by our environment, our ideas and behavior are not irrevocably determined by natural laws, immutable or otherwise." Postman, "Social Science as Moral Theology," 1988, p. 6.

24. See Bernstein, *The Restructuring of Social and Political Theory*, 1978, for a lucid introduction to the linguistic turn in philosophy.

25. Taylor, "Interpretation and the Sciences of Man," 1985.

26. Searle offers this example to illustrate the difference: "The features that an object has in virtue of which the word "dog" is true of it, i.e., the features in virtue of which it is a dog, are features that exist independently of language. . . . But the features in virtue of which today is Tuesday the 26th of October cannot exist independently of a verbal system, because its being Tuesday the 26th of October is a matter of its relations to a verbal system." Searle, *The Construction of Social Reality*, 1995.

27. Marvin Stauch expresses the distinction this way: "They [characterizations of human motivations] are, rather, creative articulations of a sense of what is desirable or undesirable—creative because, as linguistic animals, humans formulate evaluations of self and context that do not simply express descriptions of what motivates them as if these motivations were fully independent objects, that is, objects that are not altered in substance, degree, or manner, by the description." Stauch, "Natural Science, Social Science, and Democratic Practice: Some Political Implications of the Distinction Between the Natural and the Human Sciences," 1992, p. 341.

28. ". . . our articulations not only help us to define better what we want to do, they also move us. Articulating a constitutive good not only helps us fine-tune what we want to be and do, it also inspires and moves us to want to be and do it." Taylor, "Iris Murdoch and Moral Philosophy," 1996, p. 14.

29. In an elegant statement of this difference, the anthropologist Clifford Geertz writes, "Believing, with Max Weber, that man is an animal suspended in webs of significance he himself has spun, I take culture to be those webs, and the analysis of it to be therefore not an experimental science in search of law, but an interpretive one in search of meaning." Geertz, *The Interpretation of Cultures*, 1973, p. 5.

30. Taylor, "What is Human Agency?" 1985, p. 16.

31. Taylor, "What is Human Agency?" 1985, pp. 15–16.

32. Hampshire, *Innocence and Experience*, 1989, pp. 101.

33. Charles Larmore, *The Morals of Modernity*, 1996, pp. 7–8.

34. Johnson, et al., "Relative Effectiveness of Comprehensive Community Programming for Drug Abuse Prevention with High-Risk and Low-Risk Adolescents," 1990, p. 447.

35. As Yale political scientist and professor emeritus Charles Lindblom writes, "Although [natural] science may overreach itself in genetic engineering or some other heady ambition, the whole world continues to need science and engineering for one task or another: building bridges, protecting the fertility of soils, and harnessing energy among others. Not simply helpful, they are indispensable and unmistakably so. Without science and engineering, there would be no heart bypass, no moon shot, no high speed organization and retrieval of information, and no nuclear destruction. Not so for the social sciences. The centuries have given it abundant opportunities. Practiced as long as natural science, it goes back to at least ancient Greece. In the last century thousands of social scientists trying to practice methods much like those of the natural sciences have swarmed over institutions and social processes to try to extract propositions hidden to the lay mind. For all that effort and for all its presumed usefulness, I cannot identify a single social science finding or idea that is undeniably indispensable to any social task or effort. Not even one, I suggest." Lindblom, *Inquiry and Change: The Troubled Attempt to Understand and Shape Society*, 1990, p. 136.

36. Smith, "The Social Nonsciences," in *Killing the Spirit*, 1990.

37. Giddens, *New Rules of Sociological Method*, 1976.

38. Sykes, "The Pseudo-Scientists: The Social Sciences," in *Profscam*, 1988.

39. Sullivan, *Reconstructing Public Philosophy*, 1982, p. 132.

40. Angus, *Technique and Enlightenment*, 1984, p. 4.

41. Buchanan, "Reflections on the Relationship between Theory and Practice," 1994.

42. See, for example, Bandura, "Reciprocal Influence and the Limits of Social Control," in his *Social Learning Theory*, 1977. In Bandura's words, "they are uneasy about the implications of psychotechnology for programming human relations." p. 208.

43. See Chandler, Davidson, and Harootunian, *Questions of Evidence: Proof, Practice, and Persuasion across the Disciplines*, 1991.

44. Newcomb and Bentler, *Consequences of Adolescent Drug Use*, 1988, p. 60.

45. See Starr and Immergut, "Health Care and the Boundaries of Politics," 1987, p. 225: "The increased authority of science and the medical profession [have] kept health care defined as an arena of technical decision-making insulated from political contention and control."

46. Rosler and Witztum found that treating men with a testosterone-reducing drug coupled with psychotherapy produced promising results that may cure pedophilia; see Rosler and Witztum, "Treatment of Men with Paraphilia with a Long-Acting Analogue of Gonadotropin-Releasing Hormone," 1998.

47. Clarke, *Deep Citizenship*, 1996, p. 1.

48. "The overwhelming weight of evidence from research and experience on the value of participation in learning and behavior change indicates people are more committed to initiating and upholding those changes that they helped design or adapt to their own purposes and circumstances. . . . It [active participation] helps to avoid public resistance or reaction to programs that might be perceived as propagandistic, manipulative, coercive, politically or commercially directed, paternalistic, or threatening." Green and Kreuter, *Health Promotion Planning*, 1991, p. 5, 20.

49. Nietzsche, *Will To Power*, cited in Heller, *The Importance of Nietzsche*, 1988, p. 7.
50. MacIntyre, *After Virtue*, 1984, p. 12.

CHAPTER 4: IATROGENESIS IN HEALTH PROMOTION

1. Bellah, "The Ethical Aims of Social Inquiry," 1983, pp. 376–377.
2. Glanz, Lewis, and Rimer, *Health Behavior and Health Education*, 1997, pp. 28–29.
3. Hansen, "School-Based Substance Abuse Prevention: A Review of the State of the Art in Curriculum, 1980–1990," 1992.
4. According to the 1991 Barnes and Noble *New American Encyclopedia*, "Utilitarianism is a theory in moral philosophy by which actions are judged to be right or wrong according to their consequences. A dictum made famous by the utilitarian Jeremy Bentham is that an individual should seek 'the greatest happiness for the greatest number.' Utilitarianism represents an extension into moral theory of an experimental, scientific mode of reasoning because it involves the calculation of causal consequences."
5. Commenting on utilitarianism, Sullivan observes, "Judging worth by its consequences to one's own well-being has proven the most subversive philosophy ever devised." *Reconstructing Public Philosophy*, 1982, p. 63; see also, Scheffler, *The Rejection of Consequentialism*, 1982.
6. Taylor, "What is Human Agency?" 1985, p. 16.
7. Bandura, *Social Learning Theory,* 1977, pp. 4–5.
8. Bandura, *Social Foundations of Thought and Action*, 1985, p. 4.
9. Bandura, *Social Learning Theory*, 1977, p. 78.
10. Bandura, *Social Learning Theory*, 1977, p. 115.
11. Bandura, *Social Learning Theory*, 1977, p. 213.
12. Bandura, *Social Learning Theory*, 1977, pp. 58–59.
13. Bentham, *Principles of Morals and Legislation*, 1789, in J. H. Burns and H.L.A. Hart (Eds.), *An Introduction to the Principles of Morals and Legislation*, 1970.
14. Bandura, *Social Learning Theory*, 1977, p. 147.
15. Taylor, "What is Human Agency?" 1985, pp. 21–22, 36.
16. "Whereas for the simple weigher what is at stake is the desirability of different consummations, those defined by his *de facto* desires, for the strong evaluator, reflection also examines the different possible modes of being the agent. Motivations or desires do not only count in virtue of the attraction of the consummations, but also in virtue of the kind of life and the kind of subject that these desires properly belong to." Taylor, "What is Human Agency?" 1985, pp. 25–26.
17. This section is revised and adapted from Buchanan, et al., "Social Marketing: A Critical Appraisal," 1994.
18. Wiebe, "Merchandising Commodities and Citizenship on Television," 1952.
19. Kotler and Zaltman, "Social Marketing: An Approach to Planned Social Change," 1971.
20. Andreason, *Marketing Social Change*, 1995, p. 3; see also, Manoff, *Social Marketing: New Imperatives for Public Health*, 1985; Kotler and Roberto, *Social Marketing: Strategies for Changing Public Behavior*, 1989.
21. Buchanan and Wallack, "This the Partnership for a Drug-Free America: Any Questions?" 1998.
22. Buchanan and Wallack, "This the Partnership for a Drug-Free America: Any Questions?" 1998.

23. Pollay, "The Distorted Mirror: Reflections on the Unintended Consequences of Advertising," 1986.

24. Pollay, "The Distorted Mirror," 1986, p. 33.

25. Clarke, *The Want Makers*, 1989.

26. Hastings and Haywood, "Social Marketing and Communication in Health Promotion," 1991, p. 137.

27. Strausburger, "Television and Adolescents: Sex, Drugs, Rock 'n' Roll," 1990.

28. Pollay, "The Distorted Mirror," 1986, p. 18.

29. Gerbner and his colleagues have termed this phenomenon the "mean world syndrome," the more TV people watch, the deeper their mistrust of strangers. Gerbner, et al., "Growing Up with Television: The Cultivation Perspective," 1994.

30. Goldfarb, *The Cynical Society*, 1991.

31. Hastings and Haywood, "Social Marketing and Communication in Health Promotion," 1991, p. 136.

32. See Elster's chapter on "Rational Choice" in his *Nuts and Bolts for the Social Sciences*, 1989, for a representative description of this position.

33. See note 15 above.

34. Taylor, "Responsibility for Self," 1985.

35. Dumont, *From Mandeville to Marx: The Genesis and Triumph of Economic Ideology*, 1977.

36. Foege, "Public Health and Purpose in Life," 1986.

37. Ross, *Community Organization: Theory and Principles*, 1955; Alinsky, *Rules for Radicals*, 1971; Kahn, *Organizing: A Guide for Grassroots Leaders,* 1991.

38. Wartenberg, *The Forms of Power: From Domination to Transformation,* 1990, p. 12.

39. Lukes, *Power: A Radical View*, 1974, p. 11.

40. Wartenberg, *The Forms of Power: From Domination to Transformation*, 1990, pp. 23–25.

41. Israel, et al., "Health Education and Community Empowerment: Conceptualizing and Measuring Perceptions of Individual, Organizational, and Community Control," 1994, pp. 150–1. The two special issues of *Health Education Quarterly* are Volume 21, Numbers 2 and 3, 1994, edited by Nina Wallerstein and Edward Bernstein.

42. Gitlan, *The Twilight of Common Dreams*, 1995, p. 200.

43. Nietzsche, *Joyous Science*, cited in Heller, *The Importance of Nietzsche,* 1988, p. 4, emphasis in original.

44. Nietzsche, *Complete Works*, cited in Kaufman, "Nihilism,"

45. Nietzsche, *Thus Spake Zarathustra*, cited in Heller, *The Importance of Nietzsche,* 1988, pp. 4–5.

46. Heller, *The Importance of Nietzsche*, 1988, p. 10.

47. Nietzsche, *The Anti-Christ*, cited in Cecil, "Moral Values or the Will to Power," 1996.

48. See Chapter 7 on the rise of identity politics and the breakup of the Left.

CHAPTER 5: PRACTICAL REASON

1. As Stuart Hampshire notes, "This model of practical reason as deliberation, surviving from Aristotle until the present day, is still as vivid and plausible as ever." Hampshire, *Innocence and Experience*, 1989, p. 51.

2. Kenny, *Aristotle on the Perfect Life*, 1992, p. 1–2; John Searle offers a similar definition: "Practical reasoning is always reasoning about how best to decide between conflicting desires. . . . Practical reasoning differs crucially from theoretical reasoning, from reasoning about what is the case, in that practical reasoning is always about how best to decide among various conflicting desires. . . . Practical reason concerns the adjudication of conflicting desires." Searle, *Minds, Brains, and Science*, 1984.

3. Steinberger, *The Concept of Political Judgment*, 1993, p. 109.

4. Hampshire, *Morality and Conflict*, 1983, pp. 70–71. As he continues, "There are occasions of difficulty and uncertainty when I must explicitly review the considerations for and against a suggested action, and also situations where, confronting a variety of conflicting evidence or conflicting reasons, I must formulate some definite conclusion. These are occasions on which I must brood on considerations for and against, and on which salient reasons become fully explicit and present to the subject's mind, or as fully explicit as reasons ever become. . . . Practical deliberation is a process of reviewing possible future worlds."

5. Hampshire, *Innocence and Experience*, 1989, p. 18.

6. Cited in Alejandro, *Hermeneutics, Citizenship, and the Public Sphere*, 1993, p. 82.

7. Kenny, *Aristotle on the Perfect Life*, 1992, p. 2.

8. Selznick, *The Moral Commonwealth*, 1992, p. 56, 321.

9. Taylor, "Critical Notice," 1988.

10. Nussbaum, *Love's Knowledge*, 1990, p. 37, 55, 68–69.

11. Aristotle, *Nichomachean Ethics*, line 1109b23. Taylor expands, "The endless variety of situations of action meant that we could only live well if we had some kind of insightful understanding, not reducible to rules, of the requirements of virtue in each fresh context. This is what Aristotle called '*phronesis*.'" Taylor, "Justice After Virtue," 1985, p. 34.

12. Kenny, *Aristotle on the Perfect Life*, 1992, p. 91.

13. Herbert Dreyfus has pointed out that the inextricable relationship between choice and identity is one reason computers will never be able to simulate human decision-making. See, Dreyfus, *What Computers Can't Do: The Limits of Artificial Intelligence*, 1972.

14. While it would take us far astray to develop the point, it is the same Enlightenment aspiration for there to be one method that yields one and only one answer to questions that has produced the modern ethical systems of utilitarianism and Kantianism; the hope is to come up with one principle that will enable us to rank all choices hierarchically, e.g., the greatest happiness of the greatest number.

15. Nussbaum, "Non-Relative Virtues," 1993.

16. Jonsen and Toulmin, *The Abuse of Casuistry: A History of Moral Reasoning*, 1988.

17. To paraphrase T. S. Eliot, there is no method, only intelligence. See *Selected Prose of T. S. Eliot*, edited Frank Kermode, 1975, p. 55.

18. Steinberger, *The Concept of Political Judgment*, 1993, p. 11, 45.

19. Larmore, *Patterns of Moral Complexity*, 1987, p. 15.

20. MacIntyre, *After Virtue*, 1984, pp. 148–149.

21. Hampshire notes, "The rightness or wrongness of an arithmetical calculation is quite independent of the moves made in arriving at the conclusion. . . . [But] the practical conclusion of a debate on policy, whether in public or in the mind, is not similarly independent of the particular arguments which have led to the conclusion. The arguments that have led to the conclusion must be entered into the full characterization of the conclusion itself. The moral quality of the decision depends on the acceptability of the reasons: are they a sufficient justification of the actions? Therefore, practical reason requires explicit formulation of the reasons as a defense of the policy adopted." Hamp-

shire, *Innocence and Experience*, 1989, p. 52. Similarly, Bernstein remarks, "While technical activity does not require that the means that allow it to arrive at an end be weighed anew on each occasion, this is precisely what is required in ethical know-how. In ethical know-how there can be no prior knowledge of the right means by which we realize the end in a particular situation. For the end itself is only concretely specified in deliberating about the means appropriate to a particular situation." Bernstein, *Beyond Objectivism and Relativism*, 1983, p. 147.

22. Bellah, "Social Science As Practical Reason," 1983, pp. 43, 35.

23. Glanz, Lewis, and Rimer, *Health Behavior and Health Education*, 1997, p. 21.

24. Nussbaum, *The Therapy of Desire*, 1994, p. 490.

25. Taylor, Carl, "Stages of the Planning Process," 1973.

26. Anderson, *Prescribing the Life of the Mind*, 1993, p. 133.

27. Hoy and McCarthy, *Critical Theory*, 1994, p. 42.

28. Taylor, "Explanation and Practical Reason," 1995, p. 34.

29. Taylor, "Interpretation and the Sciences of Man," 1985, p. 18.

30. Appleby, Hunt, and Jacob, *Telling the Truth about History*, 1994, p. 246.

31. "In its original inspiration, discourse ethics represented a response to the value skepticism growing out of the scientistic contraction of reason to the scientific and technical domains." Rehg, *Insight and Solidarity*, 1994, p. 21.

32. Anderson, *Prescribing the Life of the Mind*, 1993, p. 11.

33. Hampshire, *Innocence and Experience*, 1989, p. 53.

34. "This is, I believe, the commonest form of practical reasoning in our lives, where we propose to our interlocutors transitions mediated by such error-reducing moves, by the identification of contradiction, the dissipation of confusion, or by rescuing from (usually motivated) neglect a consideration whose significance they cannot resist." Taylor, "Explanation and Practical Reason," 1995, p. 53.

35. Rehg, *Insight and Solidarity*, 1994, p. 28.

36. Bernstein, *Beyond Objectivism and Relativism*, 1983, p. 216, emphasis added.

37. Cited in Sandel, *Democracy's Discontents*, 1996, p. 79.

38. Cited in Steinberger, "Hannah Arendt on Judgment," 1990.

CHAPTER 6: HEALTH AND WELL-BEING

1. Ignatieff, "Modern Dying," 1988.

2. Morris, *Illness and Culture in the Postmodern Age*, 1998, p. 64; see also Baur, who writes, "In the past thirty-five to forty years Americans have concerned themselves to an unprecedented degree with their bodies, and there is a modern fascination with both health and illness. Consider our health care industry. It is the third largest industry in the country in terms of employees and third (behind construction and agriculture) in terms of incomes produced. In 1981, for example, Americans spent $247 billion, or almost 10 percent of the gross national product, on health care. Consider also the increasing popularity of television's health and hospital shows, fitness regimes, do-it-yourself doctoring books, save-your-life diets, and articles—not to mention entire magazines—devoted to the prevention of physical decline. Blood pressure kits are sold in drug stores, and wary runners can wear a ringlike device that measures and displays their heart rate. As the *Wall Street Journal* reported, 'a morbid preoccupation with death is a major component of the national scene.'" Baur, *Hypochondria: Woeful Imaginings*, 1988, pp. 133–134.

3. Barsky, "The Paradox of Health," 1988; Barsky, *Worried Sick: Our Troubled Quest for Wellness*, 1988; Knowles, *Doing Better and Feeling Worse*, 1977.

4. Callahan, "Health and Society: Some Ethical Imperatives," 1977, p. 24.

5. Kenny, *Aristotle on the Perfect Life*, 1992, pp. 1–2; see also Chapter 5 here.

6. Kekes, *Moral Wisdom and Good Lives*, 1995.

7. Dubos, *Mirage of Health*, 1959.

8. Dubos, *Mirage of Health*, 1959, p. 129.

9. Kass, "Regarding the End of Medicine and the Pursuit of Health," 1981, p. 15.

10. Kass, "Regarding the End of Medicine and the Pursuit of Health," 1981, p. 15, emphasis in original.

11. Dubos, *Mirage of Health*, 1959, p. 130.

12. Dubos, *Mirage of Health*, 1959, p. 131.

13. Wright, *The Social Logic of Health*, 1982, p. 12.

14. Susser, "Ethical Components in the Definition of Health," 1981; Englehart, "The Concepts of Health and Disease," 1981.

15. Gillick, "Health Promotion, Jogging, and the Pursuit of the Moral Life." 1984.

16. For a remarkably similar account that came out as this book was being finished, see Woolfolk, *The Cure of Souls: Science, Values, and Psychotherapy*, 1998.

17. Nussbaum, *The Therapy of Desire*, 1994, p. 49, 26.

18. Cited in Nussbaum, *The Therapy of Desire*, 1994, p. 51.

19. Kenny, *Aristotle on the Perfect Life*, 1992, p. 9.

20. Kenny, *Aristotle on the Perfect Life*, 1992, p. 15.

21. Kenny, *Aristotle on the Perfect Life*, 1992, p. 5.

22. Hampshire, *Innocence and Experience*, 1989, p. 29.

23. Aristotle, *Nichomachean Ethics*, cited in Nussbaum, *Love's Knowledge*, 1990, p. 95.

24. Taylor, "What is Human Agency?" 1985, p. 15.

25. Taylor, "What is Human Agency?" 1985, pp. 15–16.

26. Selznick, *The Moral Commonwealth*, 1992, p. 213, emphasis in original.

27. Dines and Cribb, *Health Promotion: concepts and practice*, 1993, p. 6.

28. Williams, *Ethics and the Limits of Philosophy*, 1985, p. 9.

29. Pincoffs, *Quandaries and Virtues*, 1986, p. 95.

30. Pincoffs, *Quandaries and Virtues*, 1986, p. 81.

31. Kosman, "Being Properly Affected: Virtues and Feeling in Aristotle's Ethics," 1980, p. 111.

32. Reeve, *Practice of Reason: Aristotle's Nichomachean Ethics*, 1992, p. 169.

33. MacIntyre, *After Virtue*, 1984, p. 191 and p. 187. Elsewhere, he writes, "Virtues are precisely those qualities the possession of which will enable an individual to achieve *eudamonia* and the lack of which will frustrate his movement toward that *telos*." p. 149; see also, Bellah, "The Idea of Practices in Habits," 1988.

34. See Sullivan, "Institutions as the Infrastructure of Democracy," 1995.

35. Hyland, *The Virtue of Philosophy*, 1981.

36. Nussbaum, *The fragility of goodness*, 1986, pp. 205–206.

37. Bellah, "Understanding Caring in Contemporary America," 1994, p. 28; see also the conclusion to Bellah, et al.'s, *The Good Society*, 1991.

38. Bellah, "Understanding Caring in Contemporary America," 1994, pp. 28–29.

39. Bellah, "Understanding Caring in Contemporary America," 1994, p. 33.

40. For two other thought-provoking accounts, see Langer, *Mindfulness*, 1989, and Lear, *Open-Minded: Working Out the Logic of the Soul*, 1998.

41. Fingarette, *Heavy Drinking*, 1988, p. 100–104.

42. Gerstein and Harwood, *Treating Drug Problems*, 1990; US Surgeon General's Report of Alcoholism and Alcohol Abuse, 1990.

43. As Nussbaum suggests, "To bring such diseases [of beliefs and judgment] to light . . . is a large step toward removing them." *The Therapy of Desire*, 1994, p. 34.

44. See Rowbotham, "The Women's Movement and Organizing for Socialism," 1981; and, Hartsock, "Feminist Theory and the Development of Revolutionary Strategy," 1975.

45. National Black Women's Health Project, *Self-Help Group Development As A Method To Deliver Coordinated Health Education, and Social Services*, n.d.

46. Assennato and Navarro, "Workers' Participation and Control in Italy: The Case of Occupational Medicine," 1980. I am indebted to Michael Scanlon for calling this example to my attention.

47. Assennato and Navarro, "Workers' Participation and Control in Italy: The Case of Occupational Medicine," 1980, p. 228–229.

48. Hancock and Minkler, "Community Health Assessment, or Health Community Assessment?" 1997.

CHAPTER 7: CIVILITY, TRUST, AND COMMUNITY WELL-BEING

1. Sandel, *Democracy's Discontents: America in Search of a Public Philosophy*, 1996, p. 3.

2. Sandel, *Democracy's Discontents*, 1996, p. 4.

3. Sandel, *Democracy's Discontents*, 1996, p. 5.

4. Sandel, *Democracy's Discontents*, 1996, p. 25.

5. Sandel, *Liberalism and the Limits of Justice*, 1982, p. 133.

6. Taylor, "Iris Murdoch and Moral Philosophy," 1996.

7. Taylor, "Justice After Virtue," 1985, p. 39.

8. Kekes, *Against Liberalism*, 1997.

9. Taylor, "What's Wrong with Negative Liberty," 1985, p. 227.

10. Bellah, et al., *Habits of the Heart: Individualism and Commitment in American Life*, 1985.

11. Schlesinger, *The Disuniting of America: Reflections on a Multicultural Society*, 1992; Elshtain, *Democracy on Trial*, 1995; Gitlan, *The Twilight of Common Dreams: Why America is Wracked by Culture Wars*, 1995.

12. DeMott, "Seduced by Civility," 1996.

13. DeMott, "Seduced by Civility," 1996. p. 14.

14. Goldfarb, *The Cynical Society: The Culture of Politics and the Politics of Culture in American Life*, 1991.

15. Cited in McCarthy, "Going it Alone: Americans are No Longer Joiners," 1995.

16. Putnam, "Bowling Alone: America's Declining Social Capital," 1995, p. 77.

17. Taylor, "Modes of Civil Society," 1990.

18. Havel, *The Art of the Impossible: Politics and Morality in Practice*, 1997.

19. Taylor, "Invoking Civil Society," 1995, p. 204.

20. Walzer, "The Idea of Civil Society: A Path to Social Reconstruction," 1991, p. 293.

21. Bell, *The Cultural Contradictions of Capitalism*, 1976, p. 245.

22. Shils, "The Virtue of Civil Society," 1991.

23. Cohen and Arato, *Civil Society and Political Theory*, 1995, pp. 11–12, 16, 23.

24. Walzer, "The Idea of Civil Society: A Path to Social Reconstruction," 1991, p. 294, 304.

25. Sandel, *Democracy's Discontents*, 1996, p. 27.

26. Sandel, *Liberalism and the Limits of Justice*, 1982, p. 143.

27. See Starr and Immergut, "Health Care and the Boundaries of Politics," 1987, p. 223. "But this process of politicization has been resisted precisely on the grounds that health and medicine are . . . technical matters to be resolved by professionals on the basis of scientific criteria."

28. Gadamer, *Reason in the Age of Science*, 1981, p. 77.

29. Barber, *The Logic and Limits of Trust*, 1983, p. 9.

30. Luhmann, *Trust and Power*, 1979.

31. Fukayama, *Trust: The Social Virtues and the Creation of Prosperity*, 1995.

32. Stout and Rivara, "Schools and Sex Education: Does It Work?" 1989; Moskowitz, "Preventing Adolescent Substance Abuse through Drug Education," 1983.

33. COMMIT Research Group. "Community Intervention Trial for Smoking Cessation (COMMIT): I. Cohort results from a Four-Year Community Intervention." 1995; COMMIT Research Group. "Community Intervention Trial for Smoking Cessation (COMMIT): II. Changes in Adult Smoking Prevalence," 1995; Susser, "The Tribulations of Trials— Intervention in Communities," 1995; Pancer and Nelson, "Community-Based Approaches to Health Promotion: Guidelines for Community Mobilization," 1990.

34. Sykes, "The Pseudo-Scientists: the Social Sciences," 1988; Smith, "The Social Nonsciences," 1990.

35. Burdine and McLeroy, "Practitioners' Use of Theory: Examples from a Workgroup," 1992.

CHAPTER 8: A NEW WAY OF PRACTICE

1. Minkler, "Health Education, Health Promotion, and the Open Society: An Historical Perspective," 1989, p. 20.

2. Minkler, "Health Education, Health Promotion, and the Open Society: An Historical Perspective," 1989, pp. 22–23.

3. Glanz, Lewis, and Rimer, *Health Behavior and Health Education*, 1997, p. 21.

4. Glanz, Lewis, and Rimer, *Health Behavior and Health Education*, 1997, p. 23.

5. Sullivan, *Work and Integrity: The Crisis and Promise of Professionalism in America*, 1995, p. 165–166.

6. Blumer, "What is Wrong with Social Theory?," 1970, p. 84.

7. This section is revised and adapted from Buchanan, "Beyond Positivism: Humanistic Approaches to Research and Theorizing in Health Promotion," 1998.

8. Green, et al., *Study of Participatory Research in Health Promotion,* 1995; Frankish, et al., *Participatory Health Promotion Research in Canada: A Community Guidebook,* 1997.

9. Brown, *Social Science As Civic Discourse*, 1989; Haan, et al., *Social Science As Moral Inquiry*, 1983.

10. Lindblom, *Inquiry and Change: The Troubled Attempt to Understand and Shape Society*, 1990, pp. 213ff.

11. Burdine and McLeroy, "Practitioners' Use of Theory: Examples from a Workgroup," 1992.

12. Spacks, *Boredom: A Literary History of a State of Mind*, 1995.

13. Russell, *In Praise of Idleness, and Other Essays*, 1935.

14. von Wright, *Explanation and Understanding*, 1971.

15. Anderson, *Prescribing the Life of the Mind*, 1993; Steinberger, *The Concept of Political Judgment*, 1993.

16. To reiterate, stating that people's behavior is unpredictable does not mean that it is random, inscrutable, or indecipherable. In fact, we commonly observe a fair degree of regularity in people's patterns of behavior. But that is not because these regularities are caused by a set of generalizable antecedent variables; rather, it reflects that fact that, as human beings, we share a fairly high degree of common purposes and agree on a wide range of normative expectations. See Rehg, *Insight and Solidarity*, 1994.

17. Ricoeur, *Time and Narrative*, 1983; Coles, *The Call of Stories*, 1989; Carr, *Time, narrative, and history*, 1986; Polkinghorne, *Narrative Knowing and the Human Sciences*, 1988; Sass and Woolfolk, "Truth: Narrative and historical," 1988; see also Appleby, Hunt, and Jacob, *Telling the Truth About History*, 1994.

18. MacIntyre, *After Virtue*, 1984, p. 201.

19. DeBotton expresses the point thus, "The value of a novel is not limited to its depiction of emotions and people akin to those in our own life; it stretches to an ability to describe these *far better* than we would have been able, to put a finger on perceptions that we recognize *as our own*, but could not have formulated *on our own*. DeBotton, *How Proust Can Change Your Life*, 1997.

20. Buchanan, "A Social History of American Drug Use," 1991.

21. See Jacobson, *Pride and Solace: The Functions and Limits of Political Theory*, 1978, where the pride of the title refers to the chutzpah of theorists trying to explain the meaning of life, and the solace to the comfort readers find in reading such accounts.

22. Berger and Luckman, *The Social Construction of Reality*, 1966.

23. Searle, *The Construction of Social Reality*, 1995.

24. Appleby, Hunt, and Jacob, *Telling the Truth About History*, 1994, p. 249.

25. Lindblom, *Inquiry and Change*, 1990, p. 21.

26. Anderson, *Prescribing the Life of the Mind*, 1993, p. 69.

27. Buchanan, "Building Academic—Community Linkages for Health Promotion: A Case Study in Massachusetts," 1996.

28. Rothman, "Three Models of Community Organization Practice: Their Mixing and Phasing," 1979.

29. Blumer, "What is Wrong with Social Theory?" 1970, p. 84.

30. Geertz, *The Interpretation of Cultures,* 1973.

31. Buchanan, "How Teens Think About Drugs: Insights from Moral Reasoning and Social Bonding Theories," 1991.

32. Geertz, *After the Fact*, 1995, p. 18.

33. Gitlin, "The Politics of Communication and the Communication of Politics," 1991.

34. Habermas, *On the Logic of the Social Sciences*, 1988.

35. Anderson, *Prescribing the Life of the Mind*, 1993, p. 22.

36. Freire, *Pedagogy of the Oppressed*, 1968; *Education for Critical Consciousness*, 1973.

37. Jacoby, *The Last Intellectuals*, 1987.

38. Berlin, *The Crooked Timber of Humanity*, 1991.

39. See Norris, *The Truth About Postmodernism*, 1993.

40. See Rorty, *Contingency, Irony, and Solidarity*, 1989, for example.

41. Habermas is the most well-known exponent of this position. See also Rehg, *Insight and Solidarity* (1994) and Hoy and McCarthy, *Critical Theory* (1994) for other representatives of this stance.

42. Joint Committee for the Development of Graduate Level Preparation Standards, 1997.

43. Joint Committee for the Development of Graduate Level Preparation Standards, 1997, p. 20.

44. Institute of Medicine, *The Future of Public Health*, 1988, p. 15.

45. Sullivan, *Work and Integrity*, 1995, p. 28.

46. Sullivan, *Work and Integrity*, 1995, p. 169.

47. Sullivan, *Work and Integrity*, 1995, p. 12.

48. Sullivan, *Work and Integrity*, 1995, p. 194.

49. Sullivan, *Work and Integrity*, 1995, p. 33.

50. Sullivan, *Work and Integrity*, 1995, p. 78.

51. Sullivan, *Work and Integrity*, 1995, p. 28.

52. Williams, *Making Sense of Humanity*, 1995, p. 103.

53. Green, Harvey, *Fit for America: Health, Fitness, Sport, and American Society*, 1986; Whorton, *Crusaders for Fitness: The History of American Health Reformers*, 1982; Grover, *Fitness in American Culture*, 1989.

54. Coughlin, et al., "Ethics Instruction at Schools of Public Health in the United States," 1999.

55. Pincoffs, *Quandaries and Virtues: Against Reductionism in Ethics*, 1986; for an example of this genre of textbook, see Crigger, *Cases in Bioethics*, 1993.

56. See, among others, MacIntyre, *After Virtue*, 1984; MacIntyre, *Whose Justice? Whose Rationality*, 1988; Pincoffs, *Quandaries and Virtues: Against Reductionism in Ethics*, 1986; Williams, *Ethics and the Limits of Philosophy*, 1985; Chang, *Incommensurability, Incomparability, and Practical Reason*, 1997.

57. See Hunter, *Culture Wars*, 1991, for a good example of the effort to articulate the underlying ethical assumptions in many current public debates; see also Sandel, "Moral Argument and Liberal Toleration: Abortion and Homosexuality," 1995, for another fine example of this type of analysis.

58. "For the advocate of virtue ethics, the central concern of morality shifts from determining what one is obligated to do, to determining what sort of person one should strive to be." Paul, et al., *Virtue and Vice*, 1998, p. vii.

59. Bellah, "Social Science as Practical Reason," 1983, p. 63.

60. Sullivan, *Work and Integrity*, 1995, p. 175.

61. See Pancer and Nelson, "Community-Based Approaches to Health Promotion: Guidelines for Community Mobilization," 1990; Maccoby, et al., "Reducing the Risk of Cardiovascular Disease: Effects of a Community-Based Campaign on Knowledge and Behavior," 1977; Stanford Five City Project Research Group, "The Stanford Five City Project: Design and Methods," 1985; Carlaw, et al., "Organization for a Community Cardiovascular Health program: Experiences from the Minnesota Heart Health Program," 1984; Minnesota Heart Health Program Research Group, "Community-Wide Prevention of Cardiovascular Disease: Education Strategies of the Minnesota Heart Health Program," 1986; Lefebvre, et al., "Theory and Delivery of Health Programming in the Community: The Pawtucket Heart Health Program," 1987; Lefebvre, et al., "Community Intervention to Lower Blood Cholesterol: The 'Know Your Cholesterol' Campaign in Pawtucket, Rhode Island," 1986; Puska, "Community-Based Prevention of Cardiovascular Disease: The North Karelia Project," 1984; North Karelia Project Team, "The Community-Based Strategy to Prevent Coronary Heart Disease: Conclusions from the Ten Years of the North Karelia Project," 1985.

62. Grace, "Building Community: A Conceptual Perspective," 1990.

63. This section is revised and adapted from Buchanan, et al., "The CEPA Project: A New Approach to Community-Based Program Planning," 1994.

64. Wallerstein, "Powerlessness, Empowerment, and Health: Implications for Health Promotion Programs," 1992.

65. Pretty, et al., *Participatory Learning & Action: A Trainer's Guide*, 1995; Hall and Kidd, *Adult Learning: A Design for Action*, 1978.

CHAPTER 9: JUSTICE, CARING, RESPONSIBILITY

1. Taylor, "Justice After Virtue," 1985, p. 41.

2. See, for example, Marty, *The One and the Many*, 1997; Bok, *Common Values*, 1995; Kekes, *Moral Wisdom and Good Lives*, 1995; Nussbaum, "Aristotelian Social Democracy," 1990.

3. Kekes, *Moral Wisdom and Good Lives*, 1995, p. 183.

4. Beauchamp, "Public Health As Social Justice," 1976.

5. Rawls, *A Theory of Justice*, 1971; Habermas, *Theory of Communicative Action*, 1984.

6. Taylor, "Justice After Virtue," 1985, p. 45.

7. Rawls, *The Theory of Justice*, 1971, p. 60.

8. Obviously, there are more than two points of criticism of Rawls's work, but space does not allow for a fuller discussion. Again I hope that readers will seek out the original sources.

9. MacIntrye, *After Virtue*, 1984; MacIntyre, *Whose Justice? Which Rationality?*, 1988; Taylor, "Justice After Virtue,", 1985.

10. As Taylor puts it, "The fact that this possibility doesn't even cross some people's minds is another consequence of this mistaken modern meta-ethics. A procedural ethics of rules cannot cope with the prospect that the sources of good might be plural. A single valid procedure grinds out the rules, and if it works properly, it won't generate contradictory injunctions." Taylor, "Justice After Virtue," 1985, p. 43.

11. Nagel, "Rawls on Justice," 1975, p. 10; amplifying on the same point, Pincoffs states: "It is a misleading premise because it so effectively obscures the meaning of what has a far stronger claim to be at the foundation of ethical thought: the fact that we must live with each other in as effective, meaningful, fruitful, and harmonious a way as possible. . . . What follows immediately is that tendencies within common life change through history and across cultures. . . . The cardinal sin of such [universal rule-procedural] ethical theories is that they are reductive—that they eliminate by fiat what is morally relevant and legislate the form of moral reflection." Pincoffs, *Quandaries and Virtues: Against Reductivism in Ethics*, 1986, pp. 3–8.

12. Kekes, *Moral Wisdom and Good Lives*, 1995.

13. Please note that this is distinctly different from the standard utilitarian position. The difference lies in the locus of motivation. In the description of justice provided here, individuals may be motivated to aspire to a life of integrity for a variety of reasons, *viz* relating to their sense of identity and their beliefs about what is good and right. The impetus for rewarding individuals who demonstrate integrity comes from society, as compensation for the individual's contribution to the common good. In utilitarian thought, the locus of motivation is located within the individual, who does the right thing only because of an anticipation of reward.

14. Taylor, "The Nature and Scope of Distributive Justice," 1985.

15. Taylor, "Justice After Virtue," 1985, pp. 42–3.

16. See Etzioni, *The Spirit of Community*, 1993; Etzioni, *New Communitarian Thinking*, 1995; Etzioni, *The New Golden Rule: Community and Morality in a Democratic Society*, 1996; MacIntyre, *Whose Justice? Whose Rationality*, 1988.

17. Taylor, "Justice After Virtue," 1985, p. 43, emphasis added.

18. Cited in Taylor, "Justice After Virtue," 1985, p. 42.

19. Murray, *Losing Ground*, 1984.

20. Katz, *The Undeserving Poor*, 1989.

21. Taylor, "The Scope and Nature of Distributive Justice," 1985, p. 314.

22. Phillips, *The Politics of Rich and Poor*, 1990.

23. Edsall and Edsall, *Chain Reaction: The Impact of Race, Rights, and Taxes on American Politics*, 1991; see also Hacker, *Two Nations: Black and White—Separate, Hostile, and Unequal*, 1992.

24. West, "Nihilism in Black America," 1991; and West, *Race Matters*, 1993.

25. Beauchamp, *Health Care Reform and the Battle for the Body Politic*, 1996; see also Dahl, "On Deliberative Democracy," 1997, for a thoughtful proposal for implementing such a plan.

26. Beauchamp, *Health Care Reform and the Battle for the Body Politic*, 1996, p. x.

27. The phrase "blaming the victim" is sometimes used by colleagues in a manner that suggests they believe that, because of unjust social conditions, certain groups of people cannot or should not be held accountable for their actions. I believe people are responsible for their actions; poverty does not force anyone to do anything, especially with respect to the kinds of behaviors we are talking about here—to take or not take drugs, to wear or not wear a condom, etc. But I also believe that at times people are more lucid than others about what they are trying to accomplish and many self-destructive behaviors stem from a loss of insight and clarity about the sources of their troubles, confusion about the most appropriate ways to respond to their situations, and the loss of hope that a different response would make any difference. While working to create more just social conditions, health promotion specialists might better aim to help those people become clearer about their motivations, rather than acting as apologists for inexcusable behaviors.

28. Kekes, *Moral Wisdom and Good Lives*, 1995, p. 46.

29. Bellah, "Understanding Caring in Contemporary America," 1994, p. 21.

30. Elshtain, *Democracy on Trial*, 1995, p. 14.

31. Golub, *The Limits of Medicine: How Science Shapes Our Hopes for a Cure*, 1994.

32. Phillips and Benner, *The Crisis of Care*, 1994, p. 2.

33. Hampshire, *The Age of Reason*, 1956, p. 22.

34. Lukes, *Individualism*, 1973, p. 148.

35. Lukes, *Individualism*, 1973, p. 127–128.

36. Selznick, *The Moral Commonwealth*, 1992, p. 319.

37. Phillips and Benner, *The Crisis of Care*, 1994, p. ix.

38. Fingarette, *On Responsibility*, 1967, p. 6.

39. Benner and Wrubel, *The Primacy of Caring*, 1989, p. 2.

40. "Meaning refers to the sense of value persons experience when they understand their own lives to be linked in a significant way with the larger processes at work around them. . . . To discover meaning is to find a point to living by recognizing oneself as a participant in a worthwhile enterprise whose accomplishment calls out one's energies and whose purposes define and vindicate one's having lived." Sullivan, *Work and Integrity*, 1995, p. 148.

41. Taylor, *Sources of the Self*, 1989, pp. 3–54, 91–110; as Sullivan notes, choices only become meaningful when they are perceived to possess value independent of subjective choice, distinctions of value embedded within on-going community life. Sullivan, "Institutions as the Infrastructures of Democracy," 1995.

42. Gadamer, *Reason in the Age of Science*, 1981, p. 77.

43. Gusfield, "Hey, buddy, can you paradigm?" cited in Bellah, "Social Science as Practical Reason," 1983.

References

Alejandro, Roberto. *Hermeneutics, Citizenship, and the Public Sphere*. State Universit; of New York Press, Albany, 1993.

Alinsky, Saul. *Rules for Radicals*. Vintage Books, New York, 1971.

Anders, George. *Health Against Wealth: HMOs and the Breakdown of Medical Trust*. Houghton Mifflin Company, Boston, 1996.

Andersen, Ronald, and Mullner, Ross. "Assessing the Health Objectives of the Nation." *Health Affairs*, 9(2):152–162, 1990.

Anderson, Charles. *Prescribing the Life of the Mind: An Essay on the Purpose of the University, the Aims of Liberal Education, the Competence of Citizens and the Cultivation of Practical Reason*. University of Wisconsin Press, Madison, 1993.

Andreason, Alan R. *Marketing Social Change: Changing Behavior to Promote Health, Social Development, and the Environment*. Jossey-Bass, San Francisco, 1995.

Angus, Ian. *Technique and Enlightenment: Limits of Instrumental Reason*. University Press of America, Lanham, Maryland, 1984.

Apel, Karl-Otto. *Understanding and Explanation: A Transcendental-Pragmatic Approach*. The MIT Press, Cambridge, 1984.

Appleby, Joyce, Hunt, Lynn, and Jacob, Margaret. *Telling the Truth about History*. W. W. Norton & Company, New York, 1994.

Aristotle. *Nichomachean Ethics*. Translated by Martin Ostwald. Bobbs-Merrill Educational Publishing, Indianapolis, 1962.

Assenato, and Navarro, Vincente. "Workers' Participation and Control in Italy: The Case of Occupational Medicine." *International Journal of Health Services*, 10(2):217–232, 1980.

Bandura, Albert. *Social Foundations of Thought and Action*. Prentice-Hall, Englewood Cliffs, New Jersey, 1986.

Bandura, Albert. *Social Learning Theory*. Prentice-Hall, Inc., Englewood Cliffs, New Jersey, 1977.

Barber, Bernard. *The Logic and Limits of Trust*. Rutgers University Press, New Brunswick, New Jersey, 1983.

Barsky, Arthur. "The Paradox of Health." *The New England Journal of Medicine*, 318(7): 414–418, 1988.

Barsky, Arthur. *Worried Sick: Our Troubled Quest for Wellness*. Little Brown, Boston, 1988.

Baur, Susan. *Hypochondria: Woeful Imaginings*. University of California Press, Berkeley, 1988.

Beauchamp, Dan. "Public Health as Social Justice." *Inquiry*, 12:3–14, 1976.

Beauchamp, Dan. *Health Care Reform and the Battle for the Body Politic*. Temple University Press, Philadelphia, 1996.

Bell, Daniel. *The Cultural Contradictions of Capitalism*. Basic Books, New York, 1976.

Bellah, Robert. "Social Science as Practical Reason." In Daniel Callahan and Bruce Jennings (Eds.), *Ethics, The Social Sciences, and Policy Analysis*, Plenum Press, New York, 1983, pp. 37–64.

Bellah, Robert. "The Ethical Aims of Social Inquiry." In Norma Haan, et al., (Eds.), *Social Science as Moral Inquiry*, Columbia University Press, New York, 1983, pp. 360–381.

Bellah, Robert. "The Idea of Practices in Habits." In Charles Reynolds and Ralph Norman (Eds.), *Community in America: The Challenge of Habits of the Heart*. University of California Press, Berkeley, 1988, pp. 269–288.

Bellah, Robert. "Understanding Caring in Contemporary America." In Susan Phillips and Patricia Benner (Eds.), *The Crisis of Care: Affirming and Restoring Care in the Helping Professions,* Georgetown University Press, Washington, D.C., 1994, pp. 21–41.

Bellah, Robert, Madsen, Richard, Sullivan, William, Swidler, Ann, and Tipton, Steven. *Habits of the Heart: Individualism and Commitment in American Life*. University of California Press, Berkeley, 1985.

Bellah, Robert, Madsen, Richard, Sullivan, William, Swidler, Ann and Tipton, Steven. *The Good Society*. Alfred Knopf, New York, 1991.

Belloc, Nedra, and Breslow, Lester. "Relationship of Health Status and Health Practices." *Preventive Medicine,* 1:409–421, 1972.

Bengen-Seltzer, Barbara. *Fourth Generation Managed Behavioral Health: What Does It Look Like?* Manisses Communications Group, Providence, Rhode Island, 1995.

Benner, Patricia, and Wrubel, Judith. *The Primacy of Caring: Stress and Coping in Health and Illness*. Addison-Wesley Publishing Company, Reading, Massachusetts, 1989.

Bennett, William. *The Index of Leading Cultural Indicators: Facts and Figures on the State of American Society*. Simon & Schuster, New York, 1994.

Bentham, Jeremy. Edited by James Henderson Burns and Herbert Lionel Adolphus Hart (Eds.), *An Introduction to the Principles of Morals and Legislation*, Athlone Press, London, 1970.

Berger, Peter and Luckman, Thomas. *The Social Construction of Reality*. Doubleday & Company, Inc., New York, 1966.

Berkman, Lisa, and Syme, Len. "Social Networks, Host Resistance, and Mortality: A Nine-Year Follow-up Study of Alameda County Residents." *American Journal of Epidemiology,* 109:186–204, 1979.

Berlin, Isaiah. *Four Essays on Liberty*. Oxford University Press, Oxford, 1969.

Berlin, Isaiah. *The Crooked Timber of Humanity*. Alfred Knopf, New York, 1991.

Bernstein, Richard. *The Restructuring of Social and Political Theory*. University of Pennsylvania Press, Philadelphia, 1978.

Bernstein, Richard. *Beyond Objectivism and Relativism: Science, Hermeneutics, and Praxis*. University of Pennsylvania Press, Philadelphia, 1983.

Blum, Lawrence. *Moral Perception and Particularity*. Cambridge University Press, Cambridge, 1994.

Blumer, Herbert. "What is Wrong with Social Theory?" In Norman Denzin (Ed.), *Sociological Methods: A Sourcebook*, Aldine Publishing Company, Chicago, 1970, pp. 84–95.

Bok, Derek. *The State of the Nation: Government and the Quest for a Better Society*. Harvard University Press, Cambridge, 1996.

Bok, Sissela. *Common Values*. University of Missouri Press, Columbia, 1995.

Borgman, Albert. *Technology and the Character of Modern Life*. University of Chicago Press, Chicago, 1984.

Broadie, Sarah. *Ethics with Aristotle*. Oxford University Press, New York, 1991.

Bronfenbrenner, Urie, McClelland, Peter, Wethington, Elaine, Moen, Phyllis, and Ceci, Stephen. *The State of Americans: This Generation and the Next*. The Free Press, New York, 1996.

Brown, E. Richard, and Margo, Glen. "Can the Reformers Be Reformed?" *International Journal of Health Services,* 8(1):3–26, 1978.

Brown, Richard Harvey. *Social Science as Civic Discourse.* The University of Chicago Press, Chicago, 1989.

Brown, Robert. *The Nature of Social Laws: Machiavelli to Mill.* Cambridge University Press, Cambridge, 1984.

Brubaker, Rogers. *The Limits of Rationality: An Essay on the Social and Moral Thought of Max Weber.* George Allen & Unwin, London, 1984.

Buchanan, David. "How Teens Think about Drugs: Insights from Moral Reasoning and Social Bonding Theories." *International Quarterly of Community Health Education,* 11(4):315–332, 1991.

Buchanan, David. "A Social History of American Drug Use." *Journal of Drug Issues,* 22(1):31–52, 1991.

Buchanan, David. "An Uneasy Alliance: Combining Quantitative and Qualitative Research Methods." *Health Education Quarterly,* 19(1):117–135, 1992.

Buchanan, David. "Reflections on the Relationship between Theory and Practice." *Health Education Research,* 9(2):273–283, 1994.

Buchanan, David. "Building Academic—Community Linkages for Health Promotion: A Case Study in Massachusetts." *American Journal of Health Promotion,* 10(3):29–36, 1996.

Buchanan, David. "The Relevance of Behavioral Research for Public Health Professionals." In David S. Gochman (Ed.), *Handbook of Health Behavior Research,* Plenum Press, New York, 1996, pp. 163–179.

Buchanan, David. "Beyond Positivism: Humanistic Perspectives on Theory and Research in Health Education." *Health Education Research,* 13(2):101–12, 1998.

Buchanan, David, Apostol, Edna, Balfour, Dalila, Claudio, Carmen, O'Hare, Nancy, Santiago, Carlos. "The CEPA Project: A New Model for Community-Based Program Planning." *International Quarterly for Community Health Education,* 14(4):361–377, 1993–94.

Buchanan, David and Cernada, George. "Introduction and Overview: Progress in Preventing AIDS: Dogma, Dissent and Innovation." In David Buchanan and George Cernada (Eds.). *Progress in Preventing AIDS: Dogma, Dissent, Innovation.* Baywood Press, Amityville, New York, 1997, pp. 1–17.

Buchanan, David, Hossain, Zafar, and Reddy, Sasiragha. "Social Marketing: A Critical Appraisal." *Health Promotion International,* 9(1):49–57, 1994.

Buchanan, David and Wallack, Lawrence. "This is the Partnership for a Drug-Free America: Any Questions?" *Journal of Drug Issues,* 28(2):329–356, 1998.

Burdine, James, and McLeroy, Ken. "Practitioners' Use of Theory: Examples from a Workgroup." *Health Education Quarterly,* 19(3):331–340, 1992.

Callahan, Daniel. "Health and Society: Some Ethical Imperatives." In John Knowles (Ed.), *Doing Better and Feeling Worse: Health in the United States,* W. W. Norton and Company, New York, 1977, pp. 23–33.

Callahan, Daniel. *False Hopes: Why America's Quest for Perfect Health Is a Recipe for Failure.* Simon & Schuster, New York, 1998.

Carlaw, Raymond, Mittlemark, Maurice, Bracht, Neil, and Luepker, Russell. "Organization for a Community Cardiovascular Health Program: Experiences from the Minnesota Heart Health Program." *Health Education Quarterly,* 11(3): 243–252, 1984.

Carnap, Rudolf. *Testability and Meaning.* University of Chicago, Chicago, 1956.

Carr, David. *Time, Narrative, and History.* Indiana University Press, Bloomington, 1986.

Cecil, Andrew. "Moral Values or the Will To Power." In W. Lawson Taitte (Ed.), *Moral Values: The Challenges of the Twenty-First Century.* The University of Texas Press, Dallas, 1996, pp. 37–78.

Centers for Disease Control. "Effectiveness of Smoking Control Strategies -United States." *JAMA,* 268(13):1645–1646, 1992.

Chandler, James, Davidson, Arnold, and Harootunian, Harry (Eds). *Questions of Evidence: Proof, Practice, and Persuasion across the Disciplines.* University of Chicago Press, Chicago, 1991.

Chang, Ruth (Ed.). *Incommensurability, Incomparability, and Practical Reason.* Harvard University Press, Cambridge, 1997.

Chave, Sidney. "The Origins and Development of Public Health." In Walter Holland, Roger Detels, and George Knox (Eds.), *Oxford Textbook of Public Health,* Volume 1, Oxford University Press, Oxford, 1986, pp. 3–19.

Chin, Robert, and Benne, Kenneth. "General Strategies for Effecting Change in Human Systems." In Warren Bennis, Kenneth Benne, and Robert Chin (Eds.), *The Planning of Change,* Fourth Edition, Holt, Rinehart and Winston, New York, 1985, pp. 22–45.

Clarke, Eric. *The Want Makers.* Viking, New York, 1989.

Clarke, Paul Barry. *Deep Citizenship.* Pluto Press, London, 1996.

Cohen, Jean, and Arato, Andrew. *Civil Society and Political Theory.* The MIT Press, Cambridge, 1995.

Coles, Robert. *The Call of Stories: Teaching and the Moral Imagination.* Houghton-Mifflin, Boston, 1989.

Coles, Robert. *The Call of Service: A Witness to Idealism.* Houghton Mifflin Company, Boston, 1993.

COMMIT Research Group. "Community Intervention Trial for Smoking Cessation (COMMIT): I. Cohort Results from a Four-Year Community Intervention." *American Journal of Public Health,* 85(2):183–192, 1995.

COMMIT Research Group. "Community Intervention Trial for Smoking Cessation (COMMIT): II. Changes in Adult Smoking Prevalence." *American Journal of Public Health,* 85(2):193–200, 1995.

Cook, Deborah, Guyatt, Gordon, Laupacis, Andreas, and Sackett, David. "Rules of Evidence and Clinical Recommendations on the Use of Antithrombotic Agents." *CHEST,* 102(4):305–311, 1992.

Cooper, John. *Reason and Human Good in Aristotle.* Harvard University Press, Cambridge, 1975.

Coughlin, Steve, Katz, Wendy, and Mattison, Donald. "Ethics Instruction at Schools of Public Health in the United States." *American Journal of Public Health,* 89(45):768–770, 1999.

Crawford, Robert. "Healthism and the Medicalization of Everyday Life." *International Journal of Health Services,* 10(3):365–388, 1980.

Crigger, Bette-Jane (Ed.). *Cases in Bioethics.* Second Edition. St. Martin's Press, New York, 1993.

Dahl, Robert. "On Deliberative Democracy." *Dissent,* Summer, 54–58, 1997.

Davies, John B. "Health Research: Need for a Methodological Revolution?" *Health Education Research,* 11(2):i–iv, 1996.

Dawber, Thomas, Meadors, Gilcon, and Moore, Felix. "Epidemiological Approaches to Heart Disease: The Framingham Study." *American Journal of Public Health,* 41:279–286, 1951.

DeBotton, Alain. *How Proust Can Change Your Life.* Pantheon Books, New York, 1997.

Department of Health and Social Security, *Inequalities in Health: Report of a Research Working Group.* (Chairman Sir Douglas Black), Penguin Books, London, 1980.

DeMott, Benjamin. "Seduced by Civility." *The Nation,* 263(19):11–18, 1996.

Deutsch, Claudia. "Rewarding Employees for 'Wellness'." New York *Times,* F21, September 15, 1991.

Dilthey, Wilhelm. *Selected Writings.* Cambridge University Press, New York, 1976.

Dines, Alison, and Cribb, Alan. *Health Promotion: Concepts and Practice.* Blackwell Scientific Publications, London, 1993.

Douglass, R. Bruce, Mara, Gerald and Richardson, Henry (Eds.). *Liberalism and the Good.* Routledge, New York, 1990.

Dreyfus, Hubert. *What Computers Can't Do: The Limits of Artificial Intelligence.* Harper and Row, New York, 1972.

Dubos, Rene. *Mirage of Health: Utopias, Progress, and Biological Change.* Harper and Row, New York, 1959.

Dumont, Louis. *From Mandeville to Marx: The Genesis and Triumph of Economic Ideology.* University of Chicago Press, Chicago, 1977.

Duncan, Peter, and Cribb, Alan. "Helping People Change—An Ethical Aapproach?" *Health Education Research,* 11(3):339–348, 1996.

Eakin, Joan, Robertson, Ann, Poland, Blake, Coburn, David, and Edwards, Richard. "Towards a Critical Social Science Perspective on Health Promotion Research." *Health Promotion International,* 11(2):157–165, 1996.

Eckert, Penelope. "Beyond the Statistics of Adolescent Smoking." *American Journal of Public Health,* 73(4):439–441, 1983.

Edsall, Thomas, and Edsall, Mary. *Chain Reaction: The Impact of Race, Rights, and Taxes on American Politics.* W. W. Norton & Company, New York, 1991.

Eisenstadt, Shmuel Noah. *Power, Trust, and Meaning.* University of Chicago Press, Chicago, 1995.

Elshtain, Jean Bethke. *Democracy on Trial.* Basic Books, New York, 1995.

Engberg-Pederson, Troels. *Aristotle's Theory of Moral Insight.* Clarendon Press, Oxford, 1983.

Englehardt, H. Tristam. "The Concepts of Health and Disease." In Arthur Caplan, H. Tristam Engelhardt, and James McCartney (Eds.), *Concepts of Health and Disease: Interdisciplinary Perspectives.* Addison-Wesley Publishing Company, Reading, Massachusetts, 1981, pp. 31–45.

Epp, Jake. *Achieving Health for All: A Framework for Health Promotion in Canada.* Ministry of Health and Welfare, Canada, Toronto, 1986.

Etzioni, Amitai. *The Spirit of Community: Rights, Responsibilities, and the Communitarian Agenda.* Crown Publishers, New York, 1993.

Etzioni, Amitai (Ed.). *New Communitarian Thinking: Persons, Virtues, Institutions, and Communities.* University Press of Virginia, Charlottesville, 1995.

Etzioni, Amitai. *The New Golden Rule: Community and Morality in a Democratic Society.* Basic Books, New York, 1996.

Feinleib, Manning. "New Directions for Community Interventions." *American Journal of Public Health,* 86(12):1696–1697, 1996.

Fingarette, Herbert. *On Responsibility.* Basic Books, New York, 1967.

Fingarette, Herbert. *Heavy Drinking: The Myth of Alcoholism as a Disease.* University of California Press, Berkeley, 1988.

Foege, William. "Public Health and Purpose in Life." *The Nation's Health,* January, 1986.

Frankish, C. James; George, Ann; Daniel, Mark; and Doyle-Waters, Mimi. *Participatory Health Promotion Research in Canada: A Community Guidebook*. Health Canada, Ottawa, 1997.

Freire, Paolo. *Pedagogy of the Oppressed*. The Seabury Press, New York, 1968.

Freire, Paolo. *Education for Critical Consciousness*. The Seabury Press, New York, 1973.

Freudenberg, Nicholas. "Training Health Educators for Social Change." *International Quarterly of Community Health Education*, 5(1):37–54, 1984.

Fukuyama, Francis. *Trust: The Social Virtues and the Creation of Prosperity*. The Free Press, New York, 1995.

Gadamer, Hans-Georg. *Truth and Method*. Edited by Garrett and John Cumming. New York: Seabury Press, 1975.

Gadamer, Hans-Georg. "What is Practice?: The Conditions of Social Reason." In Hans-Georg Gadamer, *Reason in the Age of Science*, translated by Frederick Lawrence, The MIT Press, Cambridge, 1981.

Gadamer, Hans-Georg. *The Enigma of Health: The Art of Healing in a Scientific Age*. Stanford University Press, Palo Alto, California, 1996.

Gambetta, Diego (Ed.). *Trust: Making and Breaking of Cooperative Relations*. Basil Blackwell, Cambridge, 1988.

Gardner, Howard. *Frames of Mind: The Theory of Multiple Intelligences*. Basic Books, New York, 1983.

Geertz, Clifford. *The Interpretation of Cultures*. Basic Books, New York, 1973.

Geertz, Clifford. *After the Fact*. Harvard University Press, Cambridge, 1995.

Gerbner, George, Gross, Larry, Morgan, Michael, and Signorelli, Nancy. "Growing Up with Television: The Cultivation Perspective." In J. Bryant and D. Zillman (Eds.), *Media Effects*. Erlbaum, Hillsdale, New Jersey, 1994, pp. 17–41.

Gerstein, Dean, and Harwood, Henrick (Eds.). *Treating Drug Problems. Volume 1*. National Academy Press, Washington, D.C., 1990.

Gerth, Hans, and Mills, C. Wright. *From Max Weber: Essays in Sociology*. Oxford University Press, New York, 1946.

Giddens, Anthony. *New Rules of Sociological Method*. Hutchinson & Company, London, 1976.

Gillick, Muriel. "Health Promotion, Jogging, and the Pursuit of the Moral Life." *Journal of Health Politics, Policy, and Law*, 9(3):369–387, 1984.

Gitlin, Todd. "The Politics of Communication and the Communication of Politics." In James Curran and Michael Gurevitch (Eds.), *Mass Media and Society*, Edward Arnold, London, 1991, pp. 329–341.

Gitlin, Todd. *The Twilight of Common Dreams: Why America is Wracked by Culture Wars*. Metropolitan Books, Henry Holt & Company, New York, 1995.

Glanz, Karen, Lewis, Frances, and Rimer, Barbara (Eds.) *Health Behavior and Health Education: Theory, Research and Practice*. Second Edition. Jossey-Bass Publishers, San Francisco, 1997.

Goldfarb, Jeffrey. *The Cynical Society: The Culture of Politics and the Politics of Culture in American Life*. The University of Chicago Press, Chicago, 1991.

Golub, Edward. *The Limits of Medicine: How Science Shapes Our Hope for a Cure*. University of Chicago Press, Chicago, 1994.

Grace, Helen. "Building Community: A Conceptual Perspective." *International Journal of the W.K. Kellogg Foundation*, W. K. Kellogg Foundation, Battle Creek, Michigan, Spring, 1990.

Green, Harvey. *Fit for America: Health, Fitness, Sport, and American Society.* The Johns Hopkins University Press, Baltimore, 1986.

Green, Jess. "Just Say No? Flirting with Suicide." *The New York Times Magazine,* September 15, 1996.

Green, Lawrence. "Modifying and Developing Health Behavior." *Annual Review of Public Health,* 5:215–236, 1984.

Green, Lawrence and Kreuter, Marshall. *Health Promotion Planning: An Educational and Environmental Approach.* Second Edition. Mayfield Publishing Company, Mountain View, California, 1991.

Green, Lawrence, George, Ann, Daniel, Mark, Frankish, James, Herbert, Carol, Bowie, William, and O'Neill, Michel. *Study of Participatory Research in Health Promotion. Review and Recommendations for the Development of Participatory Research in Health Promotion in Canada.* University of British Columbia, Vancouver, B. C., The Royal Society of Canada, 1995.

Greenwald, Peter, Cullen, Joseph, and McKenna, Jeffrey. "Cancer Prevention and Control: From Research through Applications." *Journal of the National Cancer Institute,* 79(2):389–400, 1987.

Grossman, Jerome. "Health for What? Change, Conflict, and the Search for Purpose." *Pacific Health Education Reports,* 2:51–66, 1971.

Grover, Kathryn (Ed.). *Fitness in American Culture: Images of Health, Sport, and the Body, 1830–1940.* University of Massachusetts Press, Amherst, 1989.

Haan, Mary, Kaplan, George, and Camacho, Terry. "Poverty and Health: Prospective Evidence from the Alameda County Study." *American Journal of Epidemiology,* 125(6):989–998, 1987.

Haan, Norma, Bellah, Robert, Rabinow, Paul and Sullivan, William (Eds.). *Social Science as Moral Inquiry.* Columbia University Press, New York, 1983.

Habermas, Jurgen. *Theory and Practice.* Translated by John Viertel. Boston: Beacon Press, 1973.

Habermas, Jurgen. *Theory of Communicative Action.* Translated by Thomas McCarthy. Beacon Press, Boston, 1984.

Habermas, Jurgen. *On the Logic of the Social Sciences.* The MIT Press, Cambridge, 1988.

Hacker, Andrew. *Two Nations: Black and White—Separate, Hostile and Unequal.* Charles Scribner's Sons, New York, 1992.

Hall, Bud, and Kidd, J. Roby. *Adult Learning: A Design for Action.* Pergammon Press, Toronto, 1978.

Halverson, Paul, Kaluzny, Arnold, and McLaughlin, Curtis. *Managed Care and Public Health.* Aspen Publishers, Gaithersburg, Maryland, 1998.

Hampshire, Stuart. *The Age of Reason.* Mentor Book, New York, 1956.

Hampshire, Stuart. *Thought and Action.* Chatto and Windus, Ltd., London, 1959.

Hampshire, Stuart. *Morality and Conflict.* Harvard University Press, Cambridge, 1983.

Hampshire, Stuart. *Innocence and Experience.* Harvard University Press, Cambridge, 1989.

Hancock, Trevor, and Minkler, Meredith. "Community Health Assessment, or Healthy Community Assessment?" In Meredith Minkler (Ed.), *Community Organizing and Community Building for Health,* Rutgers University Press, New Brunswick, New Jersey, 1997.

Hansen, William. "School-Based Substance Abuse Prevention: A Review of the State of the Art in Curriculum, 1980–1990." *Health Education Research,* 7(3):403–430, 1992.

Hartsock, Nancy. "Feminist Theory and the Development of Revolutionary Strategy." *Quest,* 2(2):56–77, 1975.

Hastings, Gerard, and Haywood, Amanda. "Social Marketing and Communication in Health Promotion." *Health Promotion International*, 6(2):135–145, 1991.

Havel, Vaclav. *The Art of the Impossible: Politics and Morality in Practice*. Alfred Knopf, New York, 1997.

Heller, Erich. *The Importance of Nietzsche*. University of Chicago Press, Chicago, 1988.

Hochbaum, Godfrey, Sorenson, James, and Lorig, Kate. "Theory in Health Education Practice." *Health Education Quarterly*, 19(3):295–314, 1992.

Hollis, Martin. *The philosophy of social science*. Cambridge University Press, Cambridge, 1994.

Horkheimer, Max. *Eclipse of Reason*. Continuum, New York, 1947.

Horkheimer, Max, and Adorno, Theodor. *Dialectic of Enlightenment*. Translated by John Cumming. Herder & Herder, New York, 1972.

Hoy, David and McCarthy, Thomas. *Critical Theory*. Blackwell, Cambridge, Massachusetts, 1994.

Huba, George, Wingard, Joseph, and Bentler, Peter. "Framework for an Interactive Theory of Drug Use." In Daniel Lettieri, Mollie Sayers, and Helen Pearson (Eds.), *Theories on drug abuse*. National Institute on Drug Abuse, Rockville, Maryland, 1980, pp. 95–101.

Hunter, James. *Culture Wars: The Struggle To Define America*. Basic Books, New York, 1991.

Hyland, Drew. *The Virtue of Philosophy: An Interpretation of Plato's Charmides*. Ohio University Press, Athens, Ohio, 1981.

Ignatieff, Michael. "Modern Dying: The Soul Returns to the Sickbed." *The New Republic*, 199(26):28–33, 1988.

Ingram, David. *Reason, History, and Politics: The Communitarian Grounds of Legitimation in the Modern Age*. State University of New York Press, Albany, 1995.

Institute of Medicine. *The Future of Public Health*. National Academy of Sciences Press, Washington, D. C., 1988.

Israel, Barbara, Checkoway, Barry, Schulz, Amy, and Zimmerman, Marc. "Health Education and Community Empowerment: Conceptualizing and Measuring Perceptions of Individual, Organizational, and Community Control." *Health Education Quarterly*, 21(2):141–148, 1994.

Jackson, Christine. "Behavioral Science Theory and Principles for Practice in Health Education." *Health Education Research*, 12(1):143–150, 1997.

Jacobson, Norman. *Pride and Solace: The Functions and Limits of Political Theory*. University of California Press, Berkeley, 1978.

Jacoby, Russell. *The Last Intellectuals: American Culture in the Age of Academe*. Basic Books, New York, 1987.

Johnson, C. Anderson, Pentz, Mary Ann, Weber, Mark, Dwyer, James, Baer, Neal, MacKinnon, and Hansen, William. "Relative Effectiveness of Comprehensive Community Programming for Drug Abuse Prevention With High-Risk and Low-Risk Adolescents." *Journal of Clinical and Consulting Psychology*, 58(4):447–456, 1990.

Joint Committee for the Development of Graduate Level Preparation Standards. *Standards for the Preparation of Graduate-Level Health Educators*. Society for Public Health Education, Inc., Washington, D.C., 1997.

Jonsen, Albert and Toulmin, Stephen. *The Abuse of Casuistry: A History of Moral Reasoning*. University of California Press, Berkeley, 1988.

Jonas, Hans. *The Imperative of Responsibility: In Search of Ethics for the Technological Age*. University of Chicago Press, Chicago, 1984.

Kahn, Si. *Organizing: A Guide for Grassroots Leaders.* National Association of Social Workers Press, Silver Spring, Maryland, 1991.

Kannel, William, Dawber, Thomas, Kagan, Abraham, Revotskie, Nicholas, and Stokes, Joseph. "Factors of Risk in the Development of Coronary Heart Disease—Six-Year Follow-Up Experience: The Framingham Study." *Annals of Internal Medicine,* 55(1): 33–49, 1961.

Kass, Leon. "Regarding the End of Medicine and the Pursuit of Health." In Arthur Caplan, H. Tristam Engelhardt, and James McCartney (Eds.), *Concepts of Health and Disease: Interdisciplinary Perspectives.* Addison-Wesley Publishing Company, Reading, Massachusetts, 1981, pp. 3–30.

Katz, Michael. *The Undeserving Poor: From the War on Poverty to the War on Welfare.* Pantheon Books, New York, 1989.

Kekes, John. *Moral Wisdom and Good Lives.* Cornell University Press, Ithaca, New York, 1995.

Kekes, John. *Against Liberalism.* Cornell University Press, Ithaca, New York, 1997.

Kenny, Anthony. *Aristotle on the Perfect Life.* Clarendon Press, Oxford, 1992.

Kerlinger, Fred. *Behavioral Research: A Conceptual Approach.* Holt, Rinehart & Winston, New York, 1979.

Kerlinger, Fred. *Foundations of Behavioral Research.* Third Edition. Holt, Rinehart & Winston, New York, 1986.

Kermode, Frank (Ed.) *Selected Prose of T. S. Eliot.* Faber, London, 1975.

Kipnis, David. "Accounting for the Use of Behavior Technologies in Social Psychology." *American Psychologist,* 49(3):165–172, 1994.

Klem, Mary, Wing, Rena, McGuire, Maureen, Seagle, Helen, and Hill, James. "A Descriptive Study of Individuals Successful at Long-Term Maintenance of Substantial Weight Loss." *American Journal of Clinical Nutrition,* 66:239–46, 1997.

Knowles, John (Ed.). *Doing Better and Feeling Worse.* W. W. Norton & Company, New York, 1977.

Kosman, Louis Aryeh. "Being Properly Affected: Virtues and Feelings in Aristotle's Ethics." In Amelie Rorty (Ed.), *Essays on Aristotle's Ethics,* University of California Press, Berkeley, 1980, pp. 103–116.

Kotler, Philip, and Roberto, Eduardo. *Social Marketing: Strategies for Changing Public Behavior.* Free Press, New York, 1989.

Kotler, Philip and Zaltman, Gerald. "Social Marketing: An Approach to Planned Social Change." *Journal of Marketing,* 35(3):3–12, 1971.

Labonte, Ron. "Social Inequality and Healthy Public Policy." *Health Promotion,* 1(3):341–351, 1986.

Labonte, Ron, and Robertson, Ann. "Health Promotion Research and Practice: The Case for the Constructivist Paradigm." *Health Education Quarterly,* 23(4):431–447, 1996.

Lalonde, Marc. *A New Perspective on the Health of Canadians.* Ministry of National Health and Welfare, Government of Canada, Ottawa, 1975.

Langer, Ellen. *Mindfulness.* Addison-Wesley Publishing Company, Reading, Massachusetts, 1989.

Lawson, John and Floyd, Jerald. "The Future of Epidemiology: A Humanist Response." *American Journal of Public Health,* 86(7):1029, 1996.

Larmore, Charles. *Patterns of Moral Complexity.* Cambridge University Press, Cambridge, 1987.

Larmore, Charles. *The Morals of Modernity.* Cambridge University Press, Cambridge, 1996.

Lear, Jonathan. *Open Minded: Working Out the Logic of the Soul.* Harvard University Press, Cambridge, 1998.

Lefebvre, R. Craig, Lasater, Thomas, Carleton, Richard, and Peterson, Gussie. "Theory and Delivery of Health Programming in the Community: The Pawtucket Heart Health Program." *Preventive Medicine,* 16:80–95, 1987.

Lefebvre, R. Craig, Peterson, Gussie, McGraw, Sarah, Lasater, Thomas, Sennett, Leslie, Kendall, Leigh, and Carleton, Richard. "Community Intervention to Lower Blood Cholesterol: The 'Know Your Cholesterol' Campaign in Pawtucket, Rhode Island." *Health Education Quarterly,* 13(2):117–129, 1986.

Levy, Barry. "Creating the Future of Public Health: Values, Vision, and Leadership." *American Journal of Public Health,* 88(2):188–192, 1998.

Lilienfeld, Abraham. *Foundations of Epidemiology.* Oxford University Press, New York, 1976.

Lindblom, Charles. *Inquiry and Change: The Troubled Attempt to Understand and Shape Society.* Yale University Press, New Haven, 1990.

Lofquist, William. *The Technology of Prevention Workbook.* Associates for Youth Development (AYD) Publications, Tucson, Arizona, 1989.

Luhmann, Niklas. *Trust and Power.* John Wiley & Sons, New York, 1979.

Lukes, Steven. *Individualism.* Basil Blackwell, Oxford, 1973.

Lukes, Steven. *Power: A Radical View.* The MacMillan Press, London, 1974.

Maccoby, Nathan, Farquhar, John, Wood, Peter, and Alexander, Janet. "Reducing the Risk of Cardiovascular Disease: Effects of a Community-Based Campaign on Knowledge and Behavior." *Journal of Community Health,* 3(2): 100–114, 1977.

MacIntyre, Alasdair. *After Virtue.* Second Edition. University of Notre Dame Press, Notre Dame, Indiana, 1984.

MacIntyre, Alasdair. *Whose Justice? Which Rationality?* University of Notre Dame Press, Notre Dame, Indiana, 1988.

MacIntrye, Sally. "The Patterning of Health by Social Position in Contemporary Britain: Directions for Sociological Research." *Social Science and Medicine,* 23(4):393–415, 1986.

Marmot, Michael G., Kogevinas, M., and Elston, M. A. "Social/Economic Status and Disease." *Annual Review of Public Health,* 8:111–35, 1987.

Marty, Martin. *The One and the Many: America's Struggle for the Common Good.* Harvard University Press, Cambridge, 1997.

Mausner, Judith, and Bahn, Anita. *Epidemiology: An Introductory Text.* W. B. Saunders Company, Philadelphia, 1974.

McCarthy, Abigail. "Going It Alone: Americans Are No Longer Joiners." *Commonweal,* October 20, 1995.

McCarthy, Thomas. *The Critical Theory of Jurgen Habermas.* The MIT Press, Cambridge, 1978.

McGinnis, Michael, and Foege, William. "Actual Causes of Death in the United States." *JAMA: Journal of the American Medical Association,* 270(18):2207–2212, 1993.

McKeown, Thomas. *The Role of Medicine: Dream, Mirage, or Nemesis.* Nuffield Provincial Hospitals Trust, London, 1976.

McKinlay, John, and McKinlay, Sonja. "The Questionable Contribution of Medical Measures to the Decline of Mortality in the United States in the Twentieth Century." *Milbank Memorial Fund Quarterly,* Summer, 405–428, 1977.

McKnight, John. *The Careless Society: Community and Its Counterfeits.* Basic Books, New York, 1995.

McLeroy, Ken, Bibeau, Dan, Steckler, Allan, and Glanz, Karen. "An Ecological Perspective on Health Promotion Programs." *Health Education Quarterly*, 15(4):351–377, 1988.

Miles, Matthew, and Huberman, A. Michael. *Qualitative Data Analysis: An Expanded Sourcebook.* Second Edition. Sage Publications, Thousand Oaks, 1994.

Mill, John Stuart. *Philosophy of Scientific Method.* Hafner, New York, 1950.

Minkler, Meredith. "Health Education, Health Promotion, and the Open Society: An Historical Perspective." *Health Education Quarterly*, 16(1):17–30, 1989.

Minnesota Heart Health Program Research Group. "Community-Wide Prevention of Cardiovascular Disease: Education Strategies of the Minnesota Heart Health Program." *Preventive Medicine*, 15(1):1–17, 1986.

Miringoff, Marc. *1996 Index of Social Health: Monitoring the Social Well-Being of the Nation.* Fordham Institute for Innovation in Social Policy, Fordham University, Tarrytown, New York, 1996.

Morrison, Ken. *Marx, Durkheim, Weber: Formations of Modern Thought.* Sage Publications, London, 1995.

Moskowitz, Joel. "Preventing Adolescent Substance Abuse through Drug Education." In Thomas Glynn, Carl Lukefeld, and Jacqueline Ludford (Eds.), *Preventing Adolescent Drug Abuse: Intervention Strategies*, NIDA Research Monograph, #47, DHHS Publication No. (ADM)83–1280, Government Printing Office, Washington, D.C., 1983, pp. 233–249.

Multiple Risk Factor Intervention Trial Research Group (MRFIT). "Multiple Risk Factor Intervention Trial: Risk Factor Changes and Mortality Results." *JAMA*, 248(12):1465–1477, 1982.

Multiple Risk Factor Intervention Trial Research Group (MRFIT). "Mortality Rates After 10.5 Years for Participants in the Multiple Risk Factor Intervention Group." *JAMA*, 263(13):1795–1801, 1990.

Murray, Charles. *Losing Ground: American Social Policy, 1950–1980.* Basic Books, New York, 1984.

National Black Women's Health Project. *Self-Help Group Development As a Method to Deliver Coordinated Health, Education, and Social Services.* Center for Black Women's Wellness, Atlanta, Georgia, (no date).

Nagel, Thomas. "Rawls on Justice." In Norman Daniels (Ed.), *Reading Rawls: Critical Studies on Rawls' "A Theory of Justice."* Basic Books, New York, 1975.

Nagel, Thomas. *The Last Word.* Oxford University Press, New York, 1997.

National Institute on Drug Abuse. "Drug Abuse Prevention and Communications Research." RFA: DA-98–006. Release Date: February 20, 1998.

Nelson, Andrew, Quiter, Elaine, and Solberg, Leif. "The State of Research Within Managed Care Plans: 1997 Survey." *Health Affairs*, 17(1):128–138, 1998.

Neubauer, Deane, and Pratt, Richard. "The Second Public Health Revolution: A Critical Appraisal." *Journal of Health Politics, Policy, and Law*, 6(2):205–228, 1981.

Newcomb, Michael, and Bentler, Peter. *Consequences of Adolescent Drug Use: Impact on the Lives of Young Adults.* Sage Publications, Newbury Park, 1988.

Nietzsche, Friedrich. *Thus Spoke Zarathustra.* Translated by R. J. Hollingdale. Penguin Books, London, 1961.

Norris, Christopher. *The Truth About Postmodernism.* Blackwell, Oxford, 1993.

North, Helen. *Sophrosyne: Self-Knowledge and Self-Restraint in Greek Literature.* Cornell University Press, Ithaca, New York, 1966.

North Karelia Project Team. "The Community-Based Strategy to Prevent Coronary Heart

Disease: Conclusions from the Ten Years of the North Karelia Project." *Annual Review of Public Health,* 6:147–193, 1985.

Nussbaum, Martha. *The Fragility of Goodness: Luck and Ethics in Greek Tragedy and Philosophy.* Cambridge University Press, Cambridge, 1986.

Nussbaum, Martha. *Love's Knowledge: Essays on Philosophy and Literature.* Oxford University Press, New York, 1990.

Nussbaum, Martha. "Aristotelian Social Democracy." In R. Bruce Douglass, Gerald Mara, and Henry Richardson (Eds.), *Liberalism and the Good,* Routledge, New York, 1990, pp. 203–252.

Nussbaum, Martha. "Human Functioning and Social Justice: In Defense of Aristotelian Essentialism." *Political Theory,* 20(2):202–246, 1992.

Nussbaum, Martha. *The Therapy of Desire: Theory and Practice in Hellenistic Ethics.* Princeton University Press, Princeton, New Jersey, 1994.

Nussbaum, Martha. "Non-relative Virtues: An Aristotelian Approach." *Midwest Studies in Philosophy,* 13:32–53, 1988.

Nussbaum, Martha. "Charles Taylor: Explanation and Practical Reason." In Nussbaum, Martha, and Sen Amartya (Eds.), *The Quality of Life.* Oxford University Press, Oxford, 1993, pp. 232–241.

Nyswander, Dorothy. "The Open Society: Its Implications for Health Educators." *Health Education Monographs,* 1:3–13, 1967.

Oakeshott, Michael. *On Human Conduct.* Clarendon Press, Oxford, 1975.

Ophuls, William. *Requiem for Modern Politics: The Tragedy of the Enlightenment and the Challenge of the New Millennium.* Westview Press, Boulder, Colorado, 1997.

Pancer, S. Mark, and Nelson, Geoffrey. "Community-Based Approaches to Health Promotion: Guidelines for Community Mobilization." *International Quarterly of Community Health Education,* 10(2):91–112, 1990.

Paul, Ellen, Miller, Fred, and Paul, Jeffrey (Eds.). *Virtue and Vice.* Cambridge University Press, Cambridge, 1998.

Phillips, Kevin. *The Politics of Rich and Poor: Wealth and the American Electorate in the Reagan Aftermath.* Random House, New York, 1990.

Phillips, Susan, and Benner, Patricia (Eds.). *The Crisis of Care: Affirming and Restoring Care in the Helping Professions.* Georgetown University Press, Washington, D. C., 1994.

Pincoffs, Edmund L. *Quandaries and Virtues: Against Reductivism in Ethics.* University Press of Kansas, Lawrence, Kansas, 1986.

Polkinghorne, Donald. *Narrative knowing and the human sciences.* State University of New York Press, Albany, 1988.

Pollay, Richard. "The Distorted Mirror: Reflections on the Unintended Consequences of Advertising." *Journal of Marketing,* 50:18–36, 1986.

Postman, Neil. "Social Science as Moral Theology." In Neil Postman, *Conscientious Objections: Stirring Up Trouble about Language, Technology, and Education,* Alfred A. Knopf, New York, 1988.

Pretty, Jules, Guijt, Irene, Thompson, Joun, and Scoones, Ian. *Participatory Learning & Action: A Trainer's Guide.* International Institute for Environment and Development, London, 1995.

Puska, Pekka. "Community-Based Prevention of Cardiovascular Disease: The North Karelia Project." In Joseph Matarazzo (Ed.), *Behavioral Health: A Handbook of Health Enhancement and Disease Prevention,* 1984, pp. 1140–1147.

Putnam, Robert. "Bowling Alone: America's Declining Social Capital." *Journal of Democracy,* 6(1):65–78, 1995.

Rawls, John. *A Theory of Justice*. Harvard University Press, Cambridge, 1971.

Reeve, C.David. *Practices of Reason: Aristotle's Nichomachean Ethics*. Clarendon Press, Oxford, 1992.

Rehg, William. *Insight and Solidarity: The Discourse Ethics of Jurgen Habermas*. University of California Press, Berkeley, 1994.

Ricoeur, Paul. *Time and Narrative*. University of Chicago Press, Chicago, 1983.

Rorty, Richard. *Contingency, Irony, and Solidarity*. Cambridge University Press, Cambridge, 1989.

Rosen, George. *A History of Public Health*. Expanded Edition. The Johns Hopkins University Press, Baltimore, Maryland, 1993.

Rosler, Ariel, and Witztum, Eliezer. "Treatment of Men with Paraphilia with a Long-Acting Analogue of Gonadotropin-Releasing Hormone." *New England Journal of Medicine*, 338(7):416–422, 1998.

Ross, Murray. *Community Organization: Theory and Principles*. Harper and Brothers, New York, 1955.

Rothman, Jack. "Three Models of Community Organization Practice, Their Mixing and Phasing." In Fred M. Cox, John Erlich, and Jack Rothman (Eds.), *Strategies of Community Organization: A Book of Readings*, Third Edition, F. E. Peacock, Itasca, Illinois, 1979, pp. 20–36.

Rowbotham, Sheila. "The Women's Movement and Organizing for Socialism." In Sargent, Lydia (Ed.), *Women and Revolution: The Unhappy Marriage of Marxism and Feminism*. South End Press, Boston, 1981.

Russell, Bertrand. *In Praise of Idleness, and other essays*. W. W. Norton and Company, New York, 1935.

Sandel, Michael. *Liberalism and the Limits of Justice*. Cambridge University Press, Cambridge, 1982.

Sandel, Michael. "Moral Argument and Liberal Toleration: Abortion and Homosexuality." In Amitai Etzioni, (Ed.), *New Communitarian Thinking: Persons, Virtues, Institutions, and Communities*, University Press of Virginia, Charlottesville, 1995, pp. 71–87.

Sandel, Michael. *Democracy's Discontent: America in Search of a Public Philosophy*. The Belknap Press of Harvard University Press, Cambridge, 1996.

Sass, Louis and Woolfolk, Robert. "Truth: Narrative and Historical." *Journal of the American Psychoanalytic Association*, 36:429–454, 1988.

Scheffler, Samuel. *The Rejection of Consequentialism: A Philosophical Investigation of the Considerations Underlying Rival Moral Conceptions*. Clarendon Press, Oxford, 1982.

Schlesinger, Arthur. *The Disuniting of America: Reflections on a Multicultural Society*. W. W. Norton & Company, New York, 1992.

Schwartz, Barry. *The Battle for Human Nature: Science, Morality, and Modern Life*. W. W. Norton & Company, New York, 1986.

Schwartz, Howard, and Jacobs, Jerry. *Qualitative Sociology: A Method to the Madness*. The Free Press, New York, 1979.

Searle, John. *Minds, Brains, and Science*. Harvard University Press, Cambridge, 1984.

Searle, John. *The Construction of Social Reality*. The Free Press, New York, 1995.

Seligman, Adam. *The Idea of Civil Society*. The Free Press, New York, 1992.

Seligman, Adam. *The Problem of Trust*. Princeton University Press, Princeton, New Jersey, 1997.

Selznick, Philip. *The Moral Commonwealth: Social Theory and the Promise of Community*. University of California Press, Berkeley, 1992.

Shils, Edward. "The Virtue of Civil Society." *Government and Opposition*, 26(1):3–20, 1991.

Shilts, Randy. *And the Band Played On: Politics, People, and the AIDS Epidemic*. St. Martin's Press, New York, 1987.

Silver, Allan. "'Trust' in Social and Political Theory." In Gerald Suttles and Mayer Zald (Eds.), *The Challenge of Social Control: Citizenship and Institution Building in Modern Society*. Ablex Publishing Corporation, Norwood, New Jersey, 1985, pp. 52–67.

Silver, George. "The Road from Managed Care." *American Journal of Public Health*, 87(1):8–9, 1997.

Skinner, Burrhus Frederic. *Beyond Freedom and Dignity*. Bantam/Vintage Books, New York, 1971.

Smith, Page. *Killing the Spirit: Higher Education in America*. Viking Penguin, New York, 1990.

Snow, Charles Percy. *The Two Cultures and the Scientific Revolution*. Cambridge University Press, New York, 1961.

Spacks, Patricia. *Boredom: Literary History of a State of Mind*. University of Chicago Press, Chicago, 1995.

Stanford Five City Project Research Group. "The Stanford Five City Project: Design and Methods." *American Journal of Epidemiology*, 122(2):323–334, 1985.

Starr, Paul, and Immergut, Ellen. "Health Care and the Boundaries of Politics." In Charles Maier (Ed.), *Changing Boundaries of the Political: Essays on the Evolving Balance between the State and Society, Public and Private in Europe*, Cambridge University Press, Cambridge, 1987.

Stauch, Marvin. "Natural Science, Social Science, and Democratic Practice: Some Political Implications of the Distinction between the Natural and the Human Sciences." *Philosophy of the Social Sciences*, 22(3):337–356, 1992.

Steinberger, Peter. "Hannah Arendt on Judgment." *American Journal of Political Science*, 34(3):803–821, 1990.

Steinberger, Peter. *The Concept of Political Judgment*. University of Chicago Press, Chicago, 1993.

Stout, James, and Rivara, Frederick. "Schools and Sex Education: Does It Work?" *Pediatrics*, 83(3): 375–379, 1989.

Strausburger, Victor. "Television and Adolescents: Sex, Drugs, Rock 'n' Roll." *Adolescent Medicine*, 1(1):163–191, 1990.

Sullivan, William M. *Reconstructing Public Philosophy*. University of California Press, Berkeley, 1982.

Sullivan, William. "Institutions as the Infrastructure of Democracy." In Amitai Etzioni, (Ed.), *New Communitarian Thinking: Persons, Virtues, Institutions, and Communities*. University Press of Virginia, Charlottesville, 1995, pp. 170–180.

Sullivan, William. *Work and Integrity: The Crisis and Promise of Professionalism in America*. Harper Business, New York, 1995.

Susser, Mervyn. "Ethical Components in the Definition of Health and Disease." In Arthur Caplan, H. Tristam Engelhardt, and James McCartney (Eds.), *Concepts of Health and Disease: Interdisciplinary Perspectives*, Addison-Wesley Publishing Company, Reading, Massachusetts, 1981, pp. 93–105.

Susser, Mervyn. "The Tribulations of Trials—Intervention in Communities." *American Journal of Public Health*, 85:156–158, 1995.

Susser, Mervyn, Susser, Ezra. "Choosing a Future for Epidemiology: I. Eras and Paradigms." *American Journal of Public Health*, 86:668–673, 1996.

Susser, Mervyn, Susser, Ezra. "Choosing a Future for Epidemiology: II. From Black Box to Chinese Boxes and Eco-Epidemiology." *American Journal of Public Health*, 86:678–677, 1996.

Sykes, Charles. *ProfScam: Professors and the Demise of Higher Education.* Regnery Gateway, Washington, D. C., 1988.

Syme, Len and Berkman, Lisa. "Social Class, Susceptibility, and Sickness." *American Journal of Epidemiology*, 104(1):1–7, 1976.

Tarnas, Richard. *The Passion of the Western Mind: Understanding the Ideas That Have Shaped Our World View.* Harmony Books, New York, 1991.

Taylor, Carl. "Stages of the Planning Process." In William A. Reinke (Ed.), *Health Planning: Qualitative Aspects and Quantitative Techniques.* Waverly Press, Baltimore, 1973, pp. 20–34.

Taylor, Charles. "Responsibility for Self." In Amelie Rorty (Ed.), *The Identities of Persons*, University of California Press, Berkeley, 1976, pp. 281–299.

Taylor, Charles. "What is Human Agency?" In Charles Taylor, *Human Agency and Language: Philosophical Papers, Volume 1*, Cambridge University Press, Cambridge, 1985, pp. 15–44.

Taylor, Charles. "Self-Interpreting Animals." In Charles Taylor, *Human Agency and Language, Philosophical Papers, Volume 1*, Cambridge University Press, Cambridge, 1985, pp. 45–76.

Taylor, Charles. "Interpretation and the Sciences of Man." In Charles Taylor, *Philosophy and the Human Sciences, Philosophical Papers, Volume 2*, Cambridge University Press, Cambridge, 1985, pp. 15–57.

Taylor, Charles. "What's Wrong with Negative Liberty?" In Charles Taylor, *Philosophy and the Human Sciences, Philosophical Papers, Volume 2*, Cambridge University Press, Cambridge, 1985, pp. 211–229.

Taylor, Charles. "The Nature and Scope of Justice" In Charles Taylor, *Philosophy and the Human Sciences, Philosophical Papers, Volume 2*, Cambridge University Press, Cambridge, 1985, pp. 289–317.

Taylor, Charles. "Justice After Virtue." In Michael Benedikt and Rainer Berger (Eds.), *Kritsche Methode und Zukunft der Anthropologie*, W. Braumuller, Vienna, 1985, pp. 23–48.

Taylor, Charles. "Critical Notice." *Canadian Journal of Philosophy*, 18(4):805–814, 1988.

Taylor, Charles. *Sources of the Self: The Making of Modern Identity.* Harvard University Press, Cambridge, 1989.

Taylor, Charles. "Modes of Civil Society." *Public Culture*, 3(1):95–118, 1990.

Taylor, Charles. *The Malaise of Modernity.* T. P. Verso Press, Canada, 1991. (Released in the US under the title *The Ethics of Authenticity.* Harvard University Press, Cambridge, 1992.)

Taylor, Charles. "Explanation and Practical Reason." In Charles Taylor, *Philosophical Arguments*, Harvard University Press, Cambridge, 1995, pp. 34–60.

Taylor, Charles. "Invoking Civil Society." In Charles Taylor, *Philosophical Arguments*, Harvard University Press, Cambridge, 1995, pp. 204–224.

Taylor, Charles. "Iris Murdoch and Moral Philosophy." In Maria Antonaccio and William Schweiker (Eds.), *Iris Murdoch and the Search for Human Goodness*, The University of Chicago Press, Chicago, 1996, pp. 3–28.

Terris, Milton. "The Epidemiologic Revolution, National Health Insurance, and the Role of Health Departments." *American Journal of Public Health*, 66:1155–64, 1976.

Tipton, Steven. *Getting Saved from the Sixties: Moral Meaning in Conversion and Cultural Change*. University of California Press, Berkeley, 1982.

Toulmin, Stephen. *Cosmopolis: The Hidden Agenda of Modernity*. The Free Press, New York, 1990.

Troxel, James. "The Recovery of Civic Engagement in America." In John Burbidge (Ed.), *Beyond Prince and Merchant: Citizen Participation and the Rise of Civil Society*, Pact Publications, New York, 1997, pp. 97–111.

Turner, Bryan. *Max Weber: From History to Modernity*. Routledge, London, 1992.

United States Department of Health and Human Services. *Alcohol and Health*. Government Printing Office, Washington, DC, DHHS Publication Number (ADM) 90–1656, 1990.

United States Department of Health and Human Services. *Health, United States, 1994*. Public Health Service, DHHS Publication Number (PHS) 59–1232, Hyattsville, Maryland, 1995.

United States Department of Health and Human Services. *Promoting Health, Preventing Disease: Objectives for the Nation*. US Government Printing Office, U. S. Department of Health and Human Services, Washington, D.C., 1980.

United States Surgeon General. *Healthy People: The Surgeon General's Report on Health Promotion and Disease Prevention*. General Publications Office, U. S. Department of Health, Education, & Welfare, Washington, D.C., DHEW Publication No. (PHS)79-55071, 1979.

United States Surgeon General. *Healthy People 2000*. US Government Printing Office, U. S. Department of Health and Human Services, Washington, D.C., DHHS Publication Number (PHS) 91–50212, 1991.

Verene, Donald. *Philosophy and the Return to Self-Knowledge*. Yale University Press, New Haven, Connecticut, 1997.

von Wright, Georg. *Explanation and Understanding*. Cornell University Press, Ithaca, New York, 1971.

Wallerstein, Nina. "Powerlessness, Empowerment and Health: Implications for Health Promotion Programs." *American Journal of Health Promotion*, 6(3):197–205, 1992.

Wallerstein, Nina, and Bernstein, Edward. "Introduction to Community Empowerment, Participatory Education, and Health." *Health Education Quarterly*, 21(2):141–148, 1994.

Walzer, Michael. "The Idea of Civil Society: A Path to Social Reconstruction." *Dissent*, Spring, 1991.

Wartenberg, Thomas. *The Forms of Power: From Domination to Transformation*. Temple University Press, Philadelphia, 1990.

Weber, Max. *The Protestant Ethic and the Spirit of Capitalism*. Unwin University Books, London, 1905/1930.

Weber, Max. *The Methodology of the Social Sciences*. Free Press, New York, 1949.

Weber, Max. *Economy and Society: An Outline of Interpretive Sociology*. University of California Press, Berkeley, 1978.

Weber, Max. "Science as a Vocation." In H. H. Gerth and C. Wright Mills (Eds.), *From Max Weber: Essays in Sociology*, Oxford University Press, New York, 1946, pp. 129–156.

Weed, Douglas. "Epidemiology, the Humanities, and Public Health." *American Journal of Public Health*, 85:914–918, 1995.

West, Cornel. "Nihilism in Black America." *Dissent*, Spring, 1991.

West, Cornel. *Race Matters*. Vintage Books, New York, 1993.

Whimster, Sam, and Lash Scott (Eds.). *Max Weber, Rationality, and Modernity*. Allen & Unwin, London, 1987.

Whorton, James. *Crusaders for Fitness: The History of American Health Reformers*. Princeton University Press, Princeton, New Jersey, 1982.

Wiebe, Gerhart. "Merchandising Commodities and Citizenship on Television." *Public Opinion Quarterly*, 15:679–691, 1952.

Williams, Bernard. *Ethics and the Limits of Philosophy*. Harvard University Press, Cambridge, 1985.

Williams, Bernard. *Making Sense of Humanity, and Other Philosophical Papers*. Cambridge University Press, Cambridge, 1995.

Williams, Linda. "Will to Power in Nietzsche's Published Works and the Nachlass." *Journal of the History of Ideas*, 447–458, 1996.

Wilson, William Julius. *The Truly Disadvantaged: The Inner City, the Underclass, and Public Policy*. University of Chicago Press, Chicago, 1987.

Winch, Peter. *The Idea of a Social Science and its Relation to Philosophy*. Routledge & Kegan Paul, London, 1958.

Woods, Diana, Davis, David, and Westover, Bonita. "'America Responds to AIDS': Its Content, Development, and Outcome." *Public Health Reports*, 106(6), 616–622.

Woolfolk, Robert. *The Cure of Souls: Science, Values, and Psychotherapy*. Jossey-Bass, San Francisco, 1998.

Wright, Will. *The Social Logic of Health*. Rutgers University Press, New Brunswick, New Jersey, 1982.

Wuthnow, Robert. *Meaning and Moral Order: Explorations in Cultural Analysis*. University of California Press, Berkeley, 1987.

Wuthnow, Robert. *Acts of Compassion: Caring for Others and Helping Ourselves*. Princeton University Press, Princeton, New Jersey, 1991.

Index